MW01201148

The NDRF Handbook

For Patients with

Dysautonomias

David S. Goldstein, M.D., Ph.D.
Chief, Clinical Neurocardiology Section
National Institute of Neurological Disorders and Stroke
National Institutes of Health

and

Linda Joy Smith
Founder and Executive Director
National Dysautonomia
Research Foundation
(NDRF)

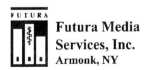

Futura Media Services, Inc.
Armonk, NY

Published by
Futura Media Services, Inc.
135 Bedford Road
Armonk, NY 10504

ISBN#: 0-913848-06-9

Made possible with a grant from the Medtronic Foundation.

The views expressed in the book do not necessarily reflect those of the US Government or National Institutes of Health.

Every effort has been made to ensure that the information in this book is as up to date and accurate as possible at the time of publication. However, due to the constant developments in medicine, neither the author, nor the editors, nor the publisher can accept any legal or any other responsibility for any errors or omissions that may occur.

Printed in the United States of America on acid-free paper.

Table of Contents

The "Automatic" Nervous System

Dysautonomias

Treatments for Dysautonomias

SECTION B: LIVING WITH DYSAUTONOMIAS 217

Foreword

Dedications

I dedicate this handbook to my family, for their support and understanding; my colleagues and friends at the NIH, for their devotion both to our research mission and to me; and especially to the many patients who have put their trust in me and provided me with sparkles of insight about how the body's "automatic" systems function in health and disease.   *--David S. Goldstein*

I dedicate this handbook to my husband and best friend, Dan, who has helped me to cope and manage my dysautonomia and become a lifeline for hundreds of individuals seeking help with this type of debilitating disorder. I also thank three of the greatest gifts God has given to me, my fantastic children Kristina, Brian, and Sarah, for their smiles, laughter, and support that keep me going. The friendship of my very dear friend Jano is unmatched by any other. I thank my sisters, Mary and Lisa, for their support. I also thank David and Suzette Levy, Frank Levine, and Dr. Lisa Benrud Larson for their contributions to this handbook, and finally my Father in Heaven—may He continue to lead me in the right direction.   *--Linda Joy Smith*

About the Authors

David S. Goldstein, MD, PhD directs the Clinical Neurocardiology Section of the National Institute of Neurological Disorders and Stroke (NINDS) at the National Institutes of Health (NIH). Dr. Goldstein graduated from Yale College and received an MD-PhD in Behavioral Sciences from Johns Hopkins. He joined the National Heart, Lung, and Blood Institute in 1978, obtaining tenure as a Senior Investigator in 1984, and in 1990 transferred to the NINDS to head the Clinical Neurochemistry Section. Since 1999 he has led the Clinical Neurocardiology Section, an independent Section in the NINDS. He has received Yale's Angier Prize for Research in Psychology, the Laufberger Medal for physiology, awarded by the Czech Academy of Sciences, and the NIH Merit Award for excellence in patient-oriented clinical research. He presided at the 8th International Catecholamine Symposium and has published more than 275 peer-reviewed journal articles and more than 70 book chapters, as well as written two single-authored academic treatises on the autonomic nervous system. His research focuses on clinical neurocardiologic disorders and catecholamine systems.

Linda J. Smith is the founder and Executive Director of the National Dysautonomia Research Foundation (NDRF). After receiving a diagnosis in 1996, Mrs. Smith and her husband established the NDRF to help fill a critical need of individuals with dysautonomia—education and support. Mrs. Smith has been an active participant in research protocols, to determine the underlying mechanisms of orthostatic intolerance, and as a lifelong patient she has become a leading spokesperson for people impacted with dysautonomia. The American Autonomic Society, the National Institutes of Health, and NASA have cited Mrs. Smith's efforts. Giving voice to over one million Americans, Mrs. Smith has worked as an advocate in the private, public, and government sectors to help raise awareness of these devastating conditions.

Introduction

> ## This book is for you.

This book is for you if you want to learn about *dysautonomias.* *Dysautonomias* are disorders of the *autonomic nervous system,* the "automatic nervous system" that regulates many body functions unconsciously, continuously, and dynamically, in everybody.

> ## Dysautonomias are disorders of "automatic" body functions.

We wrote this book for patients with *dysautonomias,* for their families and caretakers, for their doctors, and for others who seek a source of information about these disorders.

Dysautonomias range from occasional annoying sensations in otherwise healthy people to progressive, debilitating diseases. They occur in all age groups. Some are established diseases, with changes in body tissues that a pathologist can see. Some are functional disorders, with chemical or biological changes that a clinical investigator can measure. Some are mysterious and controversial, because of a lack of accepted objective tests and treatments. Some are rare and others common, but all involve more than one body function, and all have an impact on the sense of well-being. All involve multiple disciplines in medicine—cardiology, neurology, endocrinology, physical medicine, psychiatry. Predictably, relatively few cardiologists, neurologists, endocrinologists, rehabilitation medicine specialists, or psychiatrists feel comfortable in diagnosing *dysautonomias* or managing the patients.

Three factors have made the area of *dysautonomias* especially difficult.

The field of *dysautonomias* is difficult, because it is
- ## Multi-Disciplinary
- ## Integrative
- ## Mind-Body

First, the disorders are multi-disciplinary. Patients often cannot be served by specialists certified in programs in single disciplines. So one factor has been inadequate curriculum in medical schools and specialty training. Also because of the multi-disciplinary nature of *dysautonomias,* scientific peer-review committees tend to view as somewhat foreign applications for research funding and assign relatively low priority scores to the grant applications. So because of the structure of scientific review procedures, scientific research has in several ways lagged behind.

Second, the disorders are integrative. Many factors determine levels of pulse rate, blood pressure, body metabolism, pain, fatigue, and the sense of psychological well-being. These factors interact with each other, and they change over time, depending on development and circumstances of life, and they are themselves regulated as parts of complex feedback systems. Scientific theories have lagged behind, in terms taking into account this complexity.

Third—and this is where the book you are now reading comes in—*dysautonomias* are often "mind-body" disorders. Scientific theories have also lagged behind, by continuing the old philosophical distinction between physical and mental body processes. We do not believe that this is the way the body actually works, and so we do not believe that *dysautonomias* or the patients suffering with them should be classified as "medical" or "psychiatric." A major purpose of this book is educational, to teach clinicians and patients, again and again, that the many symptoms of *dysautonomias* reflect real biological or chemical changes. When clinicians cannot identify the causes of the symptoms, that ignorance should not lead to dismissing the patients as having a psychiatric rather than a "real" problem.

This book has two main sections. The first section is about what *dysautonomias* are, from the point of view of medical scientific information about normal and abnormal functions of the "automatic nervous system," diagnoses, tests, and treatments. The second section is about living with *dysautonomias*. The section emphasizes that the disorders vary greatly, the individuals suffering from them differ greatly, seemingly routine activities of daily life can produce sometimes remarkable changes in "automatic" body functions, emotional distress interacts with the disorders to produce predictable effects, treatments can have limited benefits and important side effects, and the disorders pose numerous challenges to life at home and productivity at work.

Sections of this book:
- ## What are *Dysautonomias?*
- ## Living with *Dysautonomias*

We recognize that this book will have several audiences, with very different abilities to digest the medical scientific information. This is why the book includes a large glossary of terms, with words in the text that are in italics listed in the glossary. The figures and figure legends are designed to provide a parallel text that is simpler than the main text. Each section includes text boxes, listing briefly the key points.

This book is a first attempt, and we expect it will need to be re-written repeatedly, as we receive feedback from you about its strengths and weaknesses, errors and omissions. We need to hear from you, to make sure that this book really is for you.

Let us hear from you!

You can reach the NDRF website at www.NDRF.org.

Section A: Dysautonomias

The "Automatic" Nervous System

What is the Autonomic Nervous System?

We all have a nervous system. What exactly makes up this system? What does it do? And what is the "autonomic" part of the nervous system?

This chapter is about your nervous system and how it functions when there is nothing wrong with it. You will need to understand the basics before you can understand the problems that can develop.

Your body has to be able to coordinate many different activities, just to keep you going. Some of these activities are automatic, like breathing and digesting. Some are voluntary, like moving your legs to walk across the room. Your brain uses different parts of the nervous system to regulate these activities.

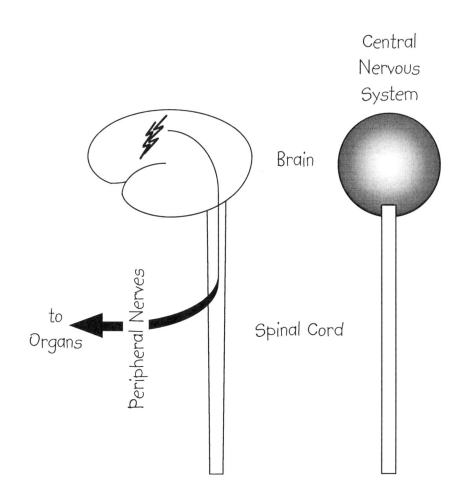

Central
Nervous
System

Brain

Peripheral Nerves

to
Organs

Spinal Cord

The central nervous system is like a lollipop on a stick. The brain is the candy. The spinal cord is the stick.

The *central nervous system* is made up of the brain and the spinal cord. The brain is like a command and control center. The spinal cord is a rope of nerves that runs from the base of your brain down through your back in your spinal column. The control signals travel from your brain to your limbs and organs by way of the *peripheral nervous system.* The *peripheral nerves* are all the nerves that lie outside the brain and spinal cord.

The *peripheral nervous system* has two main divisions. The first is the *somatic nervous system,* which helps you deal with the "outer world." The second is designed to help you regulate your "inner world," making adjustments to the systems inside your body. This is the *autonomic nervous system.*

We are going to devote the rest of this chapter to explaining the components of the autonomic nervous system and how it works.

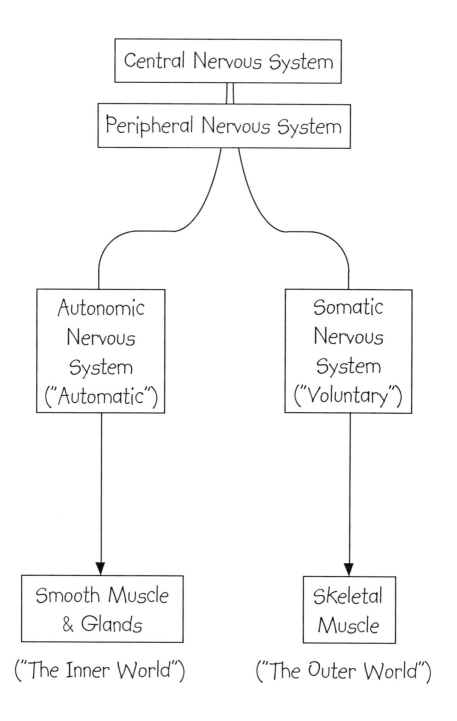

Think of the *autonomic nervous system* as the "automatic nervous system."

The *autonomic nervous system* regulates the "inner world" of the body.

The *autonomic nervous system* is responsible for many of the automatic, usually unconscious processes that keep the body going, such as...

- keeping the right **blood flow to the brain**

- keeping the right **body temperature**

- keeping the right amount of **energy production** and **fuel delivery**

- getting rid of **waste** products

- **warning signs** in dangerous situations, such as fast pulse rate, increased blood pressure, sweating, pallor, and trembling.

> *By way of the autonomic, or "automatic" nervous system, the brain controls the "inner world."*

The *autonomic nervous system* is the main way the brain regulates the "inner world." The *somatic nervous system* is the main way the body deals with the "outer world."

The autonomic nervous system sends signals to make changes to the organs in our bodies. These organs are made up of a type of muscle called *smooth muscle.* Smooth muscle is found in organs like your heart and blood vessel walls, and in your glands, such as the thyroid gland, adrenal gland, pancreas, and sweat glands. The *autonomic nervous system* sends signals to the *smooth muscle cells* that cause changes in their muscle tone. All of this happens automatically, all day and night, to keep your body functioning. The target organ of the *somatic nervous system* is skeletal muscle.

Nerves that go to skeletal muscle to regulate movement come directly from the *central nervous system*, but nerves of the *autonomic nervous system* come indirectly from the *central nervous system*, by way of clumps of cells called *ganglia. Ganglia* are like transformers on the utility pole outside your house. The transformer relays the electricity that comes in from the thick trunk lines to the thin cables that go to the house. The *ganglia* are arranged like pearls on a string along each side of the spinal cord.

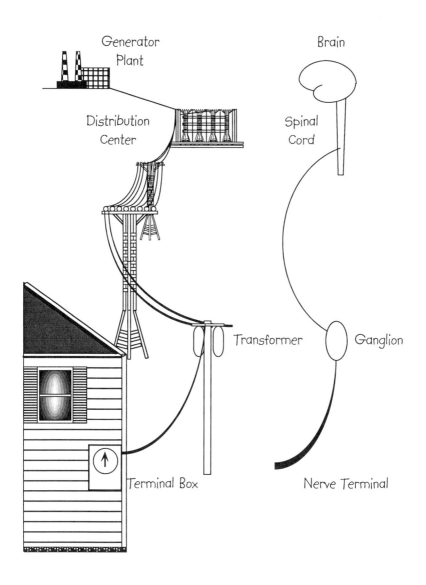

Generator Plant

Distribution Center

Transformer

Terminal Box

Brain

Spinal Cord

Ganglion

Nerve Terminal

Ganglia are like transformers that transfer the electricity from the utility pole to the terminal box outside your house.

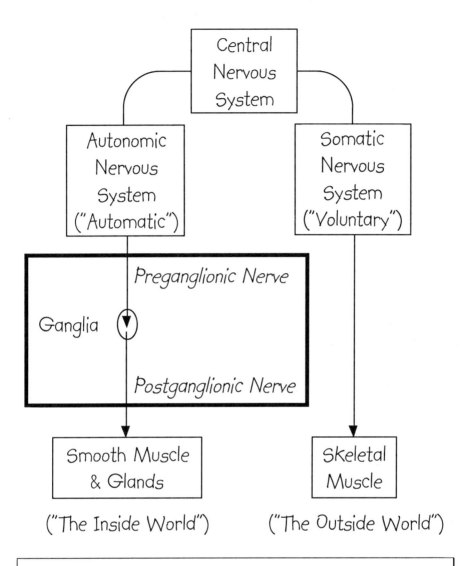

Ganglia are clumps of cells that relay control signals to the "inner world." Nerves to the ganglia are preganglionic and from the ganglia to the organs postganglionic.

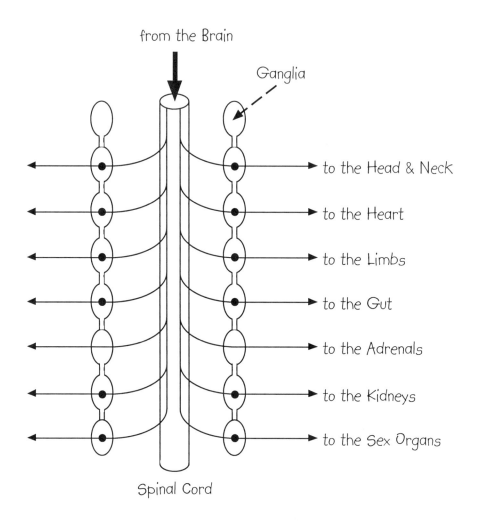

from the Brain

Ganglia

to the Head & Neck

to the Heart

to the Limbs

to the Gut

to the Adrenals

to the Kidneys

to the Sex Organs

Spinal Cord

Ganglia are arranged like pearls on a string on each side of the spinal cord.

In the *autonomic nervous system,* control signals from the brain and spinal cord go to the *ganglia* (singular *ganglion*) in the *preganglionic nerves,* and nerves from the *ganglia,* called *postganglionic* nerves, deliver those signals to the *nerve terminals* near or in the target tissues.

What are the Parts of the Autonomic Nervous System?

As first described a little over a century ago, the *autonomic nervous system* includes the *parasympathetic nervous system* and the *sympathetic nervous system.*

A third part, the relatively less well understood "enteric" nervous system, is in the gastrointestinal tract.

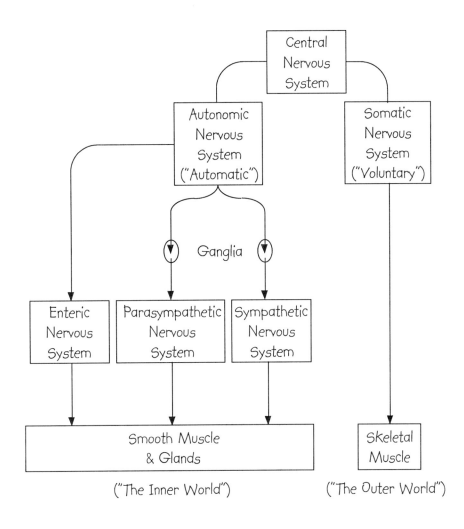

("The Inner World")   ("The Outer World")

The autonomic nervous system includes the sympathetic, parasympathetic, and enteric nervous systems, which help regulate the "inner world."

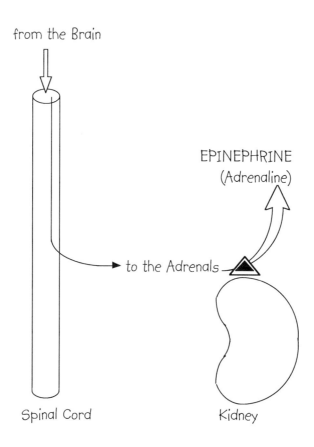

from the Brain

EPINEPHRINE
(Adrenaline)

to the Adrenals

Spinal Cord

Kidney

Epinephrine (adrenaline) is released from the adrenal glands, which sit on top of the kidneys.

Also about a century ago, the *hormone, adrenaline (epinephrine),* was discovered. *Adrenaline* is released into the bloodstream from the *medulla* (from the Latin word for "marrow") of the *adrenal glands,* which sit at the tops of the *kidneys.*

With these discoveries, scientists began to understand more about the *autonomic nervous system* and what roles it plays in our daily lives. The combination of the *sympathetic nervous system* and *adrenal glands* came to be understood as a single "emergency" system for the body. This emergency system was called the *"sympathoadrenal"* system, or *"sympathico-adrenal"* system. You may have heard of the "fight-or-flight" response that you experience in distressing situations. The *sympathoadrenal system* would help you to survive emergencies, by adjusting several body processes to enhance your ability to protect yourself (fight) or to escape (flight).

The *parasympathetic nervous system* in many ways acts like the opposite of an emergency system. "Vegetative" behaviors, activities that increase instead of use up energy, are associated with increased activity of this system. Examples of this are sleeping, eating, digesting, and excreting waste.

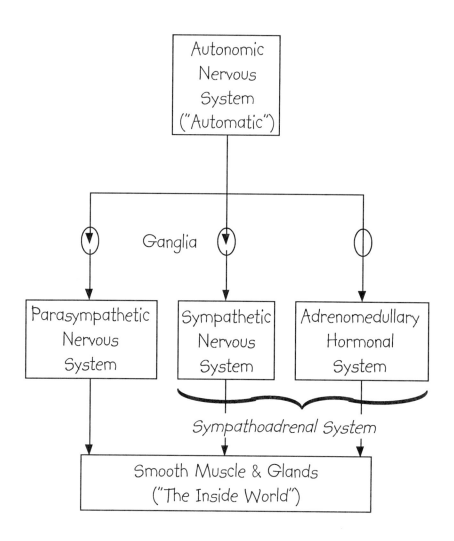

Scientists have thought the sympathetic nervous system and adrenal medulla are a single "emergency" system, the "sympathoadrenal system."

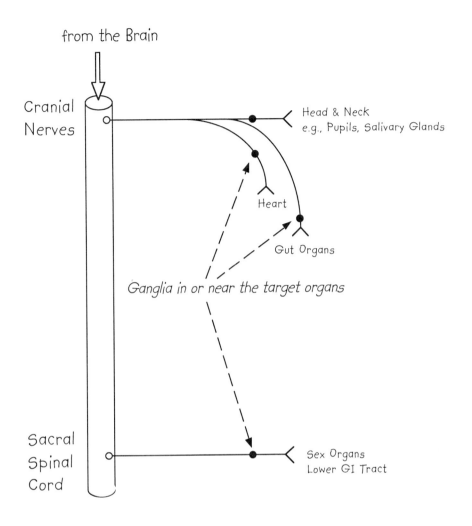

from the Brain

Cranial
Nerves

Head & Neck
e.g., Pupils, Salivary Glands

Heart

Gut Organs

Ganglia in or near the target organs

Sacral
Spinal
Cord

Sex Organs
Lower GI Tract

The parasympathetic nervous system has two parts, at opposite ends of the nervous system.

The upper part of the *parasympathetic nervous system* is the nerves that come from a portion of your brain called the *brainstem.* The *brainstem* connects the brain to the spinal cord. Most of the nerves of the *parasympathetic nervous system* come from the *brainstem.* These nerves travel to many parts of your body, including the eyes, face, tongue, heart, and most of the gastrointestinal system.

The nerves that come from the brainstem are called the *cranial nerves* (the word, "cranial," refers to the skull). The parasympathetic nerve fibers travel in major *cranial nerves* that have specific names. The *oculomotor nerve* connects to the eye, the *facial nerve* to the face, the *glossopharyngeal nerve* to the tongue and muscles involved with swallowing and talking, and the *vagus nerve* to the heart and most of the abdominal organs. You may have heard your doctor talk about some of these nerves, especially the *vagus nerve.*

The lower part of your *parasympathetic nervous system* is the group of nerves that travel from the bottom level of the spinal cord, which is called the sacral spinal cord. These nerves travel to the genital organs, urinary bladder, and lower gastrointestinal tract.

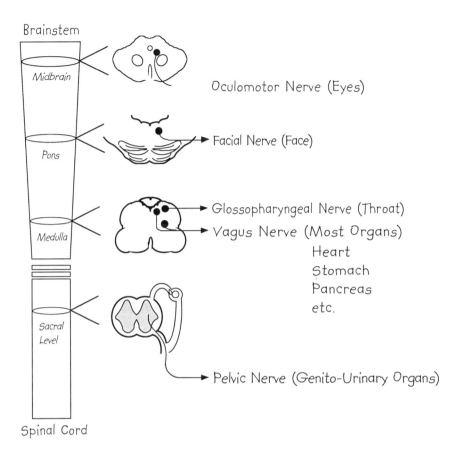

Brainstem

Midbrain — Oculomotor Nerve (Eyes)

Pons — Facial Nerve (Face)

Medulla — Glossopharyngeal Nerve (Throat)

Vagus Nerve (Most Organs)
Heart
Stomach
Pancreas
etc.

Sacral Level

Pelvic Nerve (Genito-Urinary Organs)

Spinal Cord

Parasympathetic nerves come from the brainstem and from the bottom of the spinal cord. Scientists have thought that the parasympathetic nervous system regulates "vegetative" body functions.

The nerves of the *sympathetic nervous system* come from the spinal cord at the levels of the chest and upper abdomen *(thoracolumbar spinal cord)*. The *sympathetic nerves* to most organs are *postganglionic,* coming from cell bodies in the *ganglia.* Remember that the *ganglia* are the clusters of nerve cells like a transformer on the utility pole that supplies the electricity to your house. From the prefix, "post" meaning "after," the *postganglionic nerves* come from the *ganglia,* like the electric line that comes from the utility pole to your house.

You also have sympathetic nerves that travel to your *adrenal glands* (the glands that sit on top of your kidneys and release the hormone *adrenaline*). These nerves are called *preganglionic,* from the prefix, "pre", meaning before, the *preganglionic* nerves come from cell bodies in your spinal cord and then pass through the *ganglia.* It is like a direct wiring connection from the electrical distribution center to the terminal box on your house. Most of the *sympathetic nerves* to the *adrenal medulla* are *preganglionic,* coming from cell bodies in the *spinal cord* and passing through the *ganglia.*

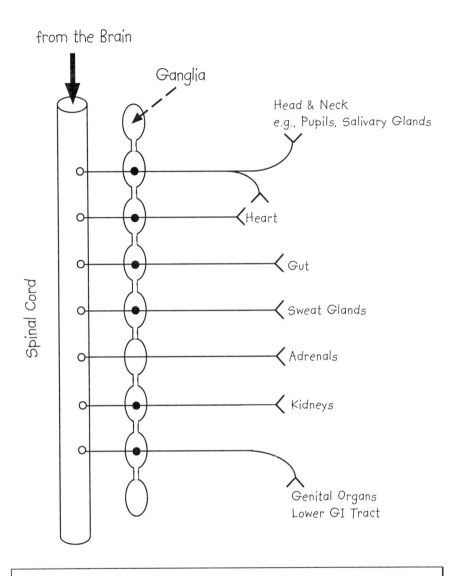

from the Brain

Ganglia

Head & Neck
e.g., Pupils, Salivary Glands

Heart

Gut

Sweat Glands

Adrenals

Kidneys

Genital Organs
Lower GI Tract

Spinal Cord

The sympathetic nerves come from ganglia attached to the spinal cord at the levels of the chest and upper abdomen.

How Does the Autonomic Nervous System Work?

The *autonomic nervous system* works by releasing messenger chemicals inside the body. These chemicals act on *receptors* on target cells, such as heart muscle cells, and this changes body functions.

For example, when you exercise on a hot day, activation of a part of the *autonomic nervous system* releases *acetylcholine,* a chemical messenger, from the nerve terminals, activating *receptors* on the cells of sweat glands. Activation of the *receptors* causes the glands to release sweat.

There are two types of chemical messengers that can be released in your body. The first type is a messenger that is released directly from the nerves in body organs. Chemicals released from nerve terminals in body organs are called *neurotransmitters.*

The second type of messenger is released directly into the bloodstream. This type of messenger is called a *hormone.* One famous *hormone* is *adrenaline,* released into the bloodstream by the *adrenal gland,* the gland that sits on top of each kidney. Chemicals released into the bloodstream are called *hormones.*

A Quick Review

Now is a good time for us to review the information so far. It can be a bit confusing, because of the several "nervous systems."

Remember, you have a *central nervous system* (your brain and spinal cord) and a *peripheral nervous system* (the rest of your nerves). Your *peripheral nervous system* has two divisions, the *somatic nervous system* and the *autonomic nervous system.* The *somatic nervous system* is concerned with the "outer world," and the nerves in this system travel to skeletal muscle. Your *autonomic nervous system* is concerned with the "inner world" of your body, and it usually works automatically, so that you can think of the *autonomic nervous system* as the "automatic nervous system."

The control signals of the *autonomic nervous system* travel indirectly from your *central nervous system* through *ganglia* (clusters of nerve cells) to *smooth muscle,* found in areas like your blood vessels, heart, and glands throughout your body. Nerves coming from the *ganglia* are called *postganglionic.* Some nerves, such as those to the adrenal glands, pass through the *ganglia* without relaying within the *ganglia,* so that there is a direct connection from the *central nervous system* to the target organs, and these nerves are called *preganglionic.*

You have also learned that there are two divisions of the *autonomic nervous system*, called the *sympathetic nervous system* and the *parasympathetic nervous system.*

And you have learned that the *autonomic nervous system* works by releasing chemical messengers that act on *receptors* located in organs throughout the body. These messengers either come from nerves *(neurotransmitters)* in body organs or are released into the bloodstream *(hormones).* The *adrenal glands* located on the tops of the kidneys are where the *hormone adrenaline* is released. The *adrenal glands,* combined with the *sympathetic nervous system*, has been called the *"sympathoadrenal system,"* which can function as an emergency system to help protect you in "fight-or-flight" situations.

Chemical Neurotransmission

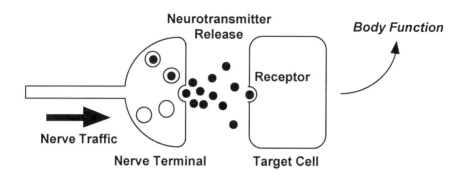

Hormone Release

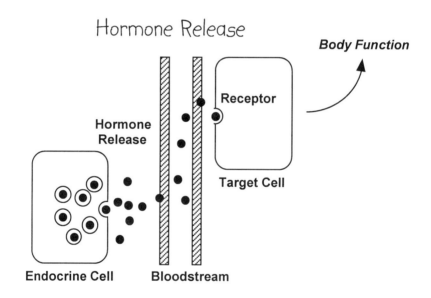

The autonomic nervous system releases chemical messengers and hormones.

What are the Chemical Messengers of the Autonomic Nervous System?

There are two main chemical messengers *(neurotransmitters)* of the *autonomic nervous system* and one main *hormone*. *Acetylcholine* and *norepinephrine* (also called *noradrenaline)* are the *neurotransmitters. Adrenaline* (also called *epinephrine)* is the *hormone* (remember that this is the *hormone* released from the *adrenal glands)*.

These chemical messengers are used differently by your autonomic nervous system. Acetylcholine (ACh) is the neurotransmitter that is used by the parasympathetic nervous system.

Norepinephrine (NE, noradrenaline) is the main neurotransmitter used by the sympathetic nervous system. Epinephrine (EPI, adrenaline) is the hormone used by the adrenomedullary hormonal system. (The adrenal medulla is the center part of the adrenal gland. It is surrounded by the adrenal cortex, which releases other hormones.)

Acetylcholine is the main chemical messenger that relays control signals from the *preganglionic* to the *postganglionic* cells in the *ganglia*. *Acetylcholine* does so by binding to a specific type of receptor called a *nicotinic receptor*. As the name suggests, *nicotine* stimulates transmission of signals within the *ganglia*.

Acetylcholine is important for "vegetative" activities, like eating, digesting, sweating, and getting rid of waste.

Acetylcholine is also used to help signal the release of *epinephrine (adrenaline)* from the *adrenal gland.* The *sympathetic nerves* that trigger the release of *adrenaline* pass through the *ganglia* and directly supply the cells in the *adrenal gland* that produce and release *adrenaline.* *Acetylcholine* is released from the *sympathetic nerve terminals* in the center of the *adrenal gland,* which is called the *adrenal medulla.* The *acetylcholine* then binds to *nicotinic receptors* on these cells, which stimulates them to release *adrenaline* into the bloodstream. The bloodstream delivers the *adrenaline* to organs throughout the body. This is how *adrenaline* is able to produce so many different effects in the body.

The bloodstream delivers adrenaline throughout the body.

We all know that cigarettes contain *nicotine.* The acute effects of *nicotine* in the body, such as fast pulse rate, increased blood pressure, sweating, and increased production of saliva, result from the release of *epinephrine* and from the increased transmission of nerve signals in *ganglia* supplying the *sympathetic nervous system* and *parasympathetic nervous system.*

The effects of nicotine in the body result from increased release of adrenaline into the bloodstream and from increased transmission of nerve impulses through the ganglia.

Norepinephrine is the main chemical messenger, or neurotransmitter, of the sympathetic nervous system.

As a *neurotransmitter, norepinephrine* released from *sympathetic nerve terminals* acts locally on nearby cells. For instance, *norepinephrine* released from *sympathetic nerve terminals* in the heart acts on heart muscle cells. A small amount of released *norepinephrine* makes its way into the bloodstream, but usually the amount is too small for *norepinephrine* to produce effects as a *hormone.* Nevertheless, specialized laboratories can measure the amount of *norepinephrine* in the bloodstream, and this can provide an index of the activity of the *sympathetic nervous system.* The chapter about testing goes into detail about the source and meaning of *plasma norepinephrine* levels.

Although the main chemical messenger of the *sympathetic nervous system* is *norepinephrine (noradrenaline),* an exception to this rule is in the sweat glands, where *sympathetic nerves* release *acetylcholine* as the signal for sweating. This means that *sympathetic cholinergic nerves* cause changes in sweating such as in response to changes in environmental temperature.

> *Norepinephrine (noradrenaline) and epinephrine (adrenaline) are in a chemical family called catecholamines.*

Catecholamines are a small family of body chemicals whose members are *norepinephrine, epinephrine,* and *dopamine. Norepinephrine* and *epinephrine* are key chemical messengers of the *autonomic nervous system.*

Dopamine is an important chemical messenger in the brain that helps to regulate movement and mood. Suprisingly, most of the *dopamine* made in the body is produced outside the brain, and the functions of *dopamine* outside the brain are still poorly understood.

You may have heard your physician talk about testing your *catecholamine* levels. This is done to help determine how your *autonomic nervous system* is working. We will talk more about this in the chapter about autonomic function testing.

What are the Functions of the Different Parts of the Autonomic Nervous System?

The *parasympathetic nervous system* regulates what are known as "vegetative" processes. These include body functions like digestion and urination. Remember that *acetylcholine* is the *neurotransmitter* used by the *parasympathetic nervous system.* *Acetylcholine* released from *parasympathetic nerves* acts to stimulate the gut, increase urinary bladder contractions, increase salivation, and decrease the pulse rate.

> *The parasympathetic nervous system regulates "vegetative" processes. The sympathetic nervous system keeps body numbers like temperature and blood pressure in check. The adrenomedullary hormonal system regulates "emergency" processes such as in distress.*

The *sympathetic nervous system* regulates unconscious "housekeeping" processes, such as tightening blood vessels when you stand up and increasing the rate and force of the heartbeat when you exercise. When you are exposed to cold, *norepinephrine* released from *sympathetic nerves* in the skin causes pallor, goosebumps, and hair standing out. The *sympathetic nervous system* therefore helps keep body numbers like temperature and blood pressure in check.

When you are exposed to heat, eat spicy foods, or experience *distress, acetylcholine* released from *sympathetic nerves* in the skin stimulates production of sweat.

The *adrenomedullary hormonal system* plays a key role in "emergencies" and *"distress,"* when all organs of the body are threatened, such as by low blood sugar *(hypoglycemia),* low blood temperature *(hypothermia),* choking *(asphyxiation),* shock, and fear. *Adrenaline* increases blood *glucose* levels, increases pulse rate and blood pressure, stimulates metabolism, quiets the gut, and dilates blood vessels in skeletal muscle.

Psychologists and researchers have differed about the meanings of *"stress"* and *"distress"* as medical scientific ideas. For the purposes of this book, *"stress"* is a condition where the brain senses a challenge to physical or mental stability that leads to altered activity of systems to meet that challenge; and *"distress"* is a form of *stress* where there is a sense that you can't cope with the situation, you want to avoid or escape it, you show built-in, instinctively communicated signs, and the *adrenal gland* is activated. According to these definitions, neither *stress* nor *distress* is necessarily harmful or causes disease.

Sympathetic   Parasympathetic

↑ Pulse rate   ↓ Pulse rate

↓ Gut tone   ↑ Gut tone

↓ Bladder tone   ↑ Bladder tone

Dilated pupils   Constricted pupils

...but not always...

Sympathetic   Parasympathetic

↑ Saliva (thick)   ↑ Saliva (mucus)

Ejaculation   Erection

The Sympathetic Norepinephrine System and the Adrenomedullary Hormonal System usually work together,

	SNS	**AHS**
Pulse rate	↑	↑
Systolic blood pressure	↑	↑
Gut tone	↓	↓
Sweating	↑	↑
Dilated pupils	↑	↑

...but not always...

	SNS	**AHS**
Periph. resistance	↑	↓
Skeletal m. blood flow	↓	↑
Fainting	↓	↑

Parasympathetic Acetylcholine Effects

- Decreased pulse rate
- Increased salivation (watery)
- Stimulation of the gut
- Stimulation of the urinary bladder
- Penile erection
- Constriction of the pupils

Sympathetic Norepinephrine Effects

- Tightens blood vessels ⎤
- Increased pulse rate ⎬ Increased blood pressure
- Increased force of heartbeat ⎦
- Relaxation of the gut
- Emotional sweating
- Goosebumps and hair standing out
- Salt retention by the kidneys
- Increased salivation (mucus)
- Dilation of the pupils

Sympathetic Acetycholine Effects

- Sweating from altered temperature
- Sweating from eating spicy foods

Adrenomedullary Hormonal Effects

- Increased pulse rate
- Increased force of heartbeat
- Constriction of skin blood vessels (pallor)
- Dilation of the pupils
- Relaxation of the gut
- Increased blood sugar
- Decreased serum potassium level
- Increased respiration
- Emotional sweating
- Anti-fatigue effect
- Increased emotional intensity

Summing Up

You now have a basic understanding of your *autonomic nervous system.* It plays a critical role both in emergencies and in our daily activities, working to keep us going and helping our bodies make adjustments throughout the day.

Much of what you have learned may seem a bit complicated, but if you remember the basics, this will help you understand what can happen in your body if the *autonomic nervous system* is not working like it should.

You will probably need to refer back to this chapter for review as you continue to learn about the disorders and testing of the *autonomic nervous system* and the treatments of *dysautonomias* in the following chapters.

What are Dysautonomias?

Dysautonomias are conditions where altered activity of the *"automatic" nervous system (the autonomic nervous system)* is harmful to health.

In Dysautonomias, What Goes Wrong?

Probably the most common type of *dysautonomia* is a condition where altered *autonomic nervous system* function worsens another disease process that happens to be going on at the same time. For instance, when a person shovels snow, the exercise and cold exposure while standing up activate the *sympathetic nervous system*, and this increases the blood pressure, pulse rate, and the force of the heartbeat, which are appropriate responses. More blood is delivered to the heart muscle, which uses up oxygen because of the increased work of the heart. But if the person has severe *coronary artery disease*, where the blood vessels that are supposed to deliver blood to the heart muscle are narrowed, the blood supply does not increase to meet the increased demand for oxygen. This imbalance can lead to a heart attack or fatal abnormal heart rhythm. In other words, in this situation, the increased sympathetic nervous system outflow would be appropriate, but the person ends up suffering anyway, because of the worsening of an independent disease.

In other forms of *dysautonomia*, the problem is from abnormal function of the *autonomic nervous system* itself. This is the form of *dysautonomia* that most of the rest of this book is about.

> *Altered "automatic" nervous system function can worsen another disease or can itself harm health. In this book, "dysautonomias" refer to disorders of the autonomic nervous system itself.*

For a variety of reasons, we know much more about what goes wrong with the *sympathetic nervous system* than with other parts of the *autonomic nervous system* in *dysautonomias*.

In general, there are two ways *dysautonomias* can result from abnormal function of the *sympathetic nervous system*. The first is when the system is activated to take over when another system fails. We call this compensatory activation. The second is when there is a primary abnormality of the system.

Finally, there are two general ways the function of the *sympathetic nervous system* can be abnormal. The first is by underactivity of the system, and the second is overactivity of the system. Both underactivity and overactivity of the *sympathetic nervous system* can be persistent and long-term or can be occasional and short-term—in other words, chronic or episodic.

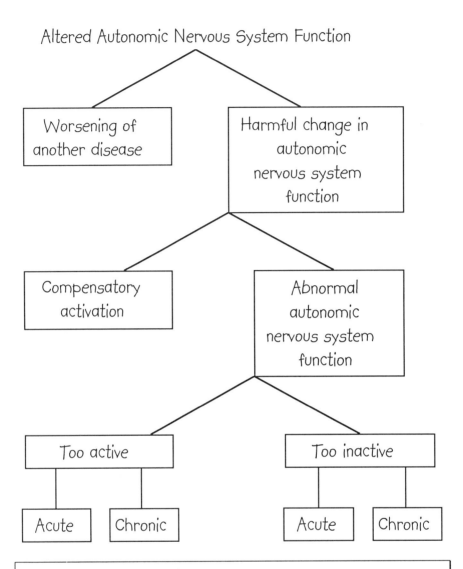

Altered Autonomic Nervous System Function

Worsening of another disease

Harmful change in autonomic nervous system function

Compensatory activation

Abnormal autonomic nervous system function

Too active

Acute

Chronic

Too inactive

Acute

Chronic

There are four types of dysautonomia, depending on whether there is too much or too little activity and whether the condition is new or has been going on a long time.

The "Mind-Body" Issue

It is worthwhile to discuss here the issue of the "mind versus body" as a primary cause of disease, because *dysautonomias* are, possibly more than any other ailments, mind-body disorders.

> *Dysautonomias are mind-body disorders.*

This is a difficult subject for both doctors and patients. The problem is the old notion that the body and mind are separate and distinct in a person, and so diseases must be either physical or mental. If the disorder were physical, it would be "real," something imposed on the individual, while if it were mental, and "in your head," it would not be real, but something created in and by the individual.

Mind ⟶ Thoughts ⟶ Mental Illness

Body ⟶ Imposed Challenges ⟶ Physical Illness

> *Traditional separation of mental from physical illness.*

> *Distinctions between the "body" and the "mind," the physical and mental, problems imposed on the individual and those in the mind of the individual, are unhelpful in trying to understand dysautonomias.*

These notions date from the teachings of the Renaissance philosopher, Descartes. They are outdated by now and also inappropriate and unhelpful in trying to understand disorders of the *autonomic nervous system.*

Here is why. Remember in the first chapter you learned about the "inner world" and the "outer world"? The mind deals with both worlds, simultaneously, continuously, and dynamically in life. Conversely, both worlds affect the mind, and each individual filters and colors perceptions of the inner and outer world. For instance, there is no such thing as a person exercising without "central command," to tense and relax specific muscles. At the same time, and as part of the same process, the brain automatically directs changes in blood flow to the muscles. The exercising muscle and changes in blood flow lead to information—feedback—to the brain about how things are going both outside and inside the body.

> *The autonomic nervous system operates at the border of the mind and body.*

Now here is the key: The *autonomic nervous system* operates exactly at the border of the mind and body. The brain uses and depends on the *autonomic nervous system* for the internal adjustments that accompany every motion a person performs and every emotion a person feels.

You already know this, if you think about it. When you jog, for instance, the blood flow to the skin and muscle increases, the heart pumps more blood, you sweat, and you move more air. These are automatic features of the experience of exercising. Can you imagine exercising and not noticing these things?

It's also true that virtually every emotion a person feels includes changes in the same body functions. For instance, when you are enraged, the blood flow to the skin and muscle increases, the heart pumps more blood, you sweat, and you move more air.

From the point of view of the bodily changes, it would matter little whether these changes resulted from the physical experience of exercise or the mental experience of rage. Both situations involve alterations in the activity of components of the *autonomic nervous system.* Both

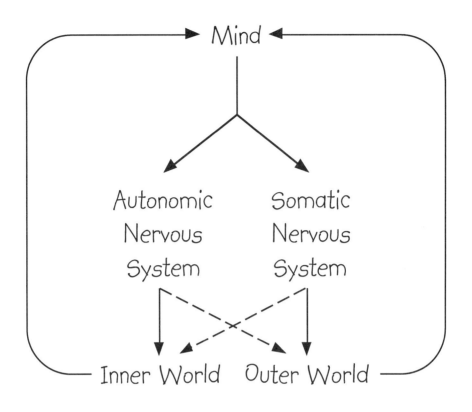

A systems approach to the mind-body issue.

situations involve changes in the inner and outer worlds. And if your *autonomic nervous system* were to malfunction, your reactions to **either** situation would not be regulated correctly, in either situation you could feel sick, look sick, and *be* sick!

A "systems" approach helps to understand *dysautonomias.* According to the systems approach, the mind simultaneously directs changes in the *somatic nervous system* and the *autonomic nervous system,* based on perceptions about what is going on in the inner world and the outer world.

Note that the *autonomic nervous system* affects both the inner world and outer worlds. For instance, if a person looked pale, because the blood quite literally had drained from the face, and was sweaty, trembling, and mumbling incoherently, other people would likely react to these signs of distress and ask, "Are you OK?" And it is well known that strong emotions, probably via *adrenaline* release, can energize an individual. In fact, one of the entries under weightlifting in the Guiness Book of Records referred to a 123-pound mother who summoned the strength to lift the front end of a 3,600-pound car after a jack had collapsed and the car had fallen on her child!

Analogously, the *somatic nervous system* can affect the inner world. For instance, you can voluntarily increase your blood pressure any time you want, by clenching a tight fist, or dunking your hand in cold water.

How would a systems approach help to understand a *dysautonomia?* A malfunction at almost any part of the system could lead to an alteration in activity of the *autonomic nervous system.* For instance, if there were no feedback to the brain about the state of the blood pressure (part of the inner world), then there would be an inability to keep the blood pressure within bounds, by changing the activity of the *autonomic nervous system.* If there were no feedback about the extent of physical exercise, there would also be an inability to adjust the blood pressure and blood flows appropriately. Of course, if there were a failure of the *autonomic nervous system* itself, this would also interfere with regulation of the inner world, but there would also be difficulty in dealing with the outer world, manifested by problems like exercise intolerance or an inability to tolerate standing for a prolonged period *(orthostatic intolerance)*. Finally, if the person had a psychiatric disorder such as panic/anxiety, then the inappropriate emotional experience of fear would be linked to both *autonomic nervous system* and *somatic nervous system* changes.

A clinician's ability to treat a *dysautonomia* successfully would also benefit from a systems approach. Treatments at any of several steps might help, but the best place in the system to insert a treatment would be the step closest to where the problem is.

When in Life do Dysautonomias Occur?

Different types of *dysautonomia* occur in different stages of life.

Dysautonomias can occur at any age.

In infants and children, *dysautonomia* often reflects a genetic change, called a *mutation*. A mutation is like a "typo" in the genetic encyclopedia.

One type of mutation that runs in the family of people of east European Jewish extraction causes *familial dysautonomia*. Another *mutation* that produces *dysautonomias* in children causes a type of phenylketonuria (PKU). Another causes "kinky hair disease" (Menkes disease). In general, *dysautonomias* from genetic *mutations* are rare. In adults, *dysautonomia*

Infancy/Childhood

Sensory and Autonomic Neuropathy (SAN)
Familial Dysautonomia (a form of SAN)
Menkes Disease

Childhood/Adulthood

Postural Tachycardia Syndrome (POTS)
Neurocardiogenic Syncope (NCS)
Hypernoradrenergic Hypertension
Autoimmune Autonomic Failure
Acute Baroreflex Failure

Adulthood/Elderly

Diabetic Autonomic Neuropathy
Chemotherapy
Parkinson's Disease
Amyloidosis
Multiple Myeloma
Multiple System Atrophy (MSA)
Shy-Drager Syndrome (a form of MSA)
Pure Autonomic Failure (PAF)

Different forms of dysautonomia happen at different ages. Here are some examples.

usually reflects a functional change in a generally intact *autonomic nervous system.*

Examples are *neurocardiogenic syncope* (where the person has frequent episodes of fainting or near-fainting), *postural tachycardia syndrome* (where the person cannot tolerate standing up for long periods and has a rapid pulse rate during standing), and *hypernoradrenergic hypertension* (where overactivity of the *sympathetic nervous system* causes a form of high blood pressure). Less commonly, there is a loss of nerve terminals, such as caused by a toxic substance, viral infection, or the body attacking itself (*autoimmune autonomic failure*). Rarely, *dysautonomia* in adults reflects a genetic *mutation*, the one-in-a-million "typo" in the genetic encyclopedia, or a *polymorphism*, which is genetic change that is more common than a *mutation.*

In the elderly, *dysautonomia* usually reflects a degeneration of the *autonomic nervous system*, often in assocation with other evidence of degeneration of the brain. Examples are *multiple system atrophy* and *Parkinson's disease.*

How Are Dysautonomias Classified?

Since *dysautonomias* can be somewhat mysterious and controversial, doctors can disagree about the diagnostic classification of *dysautonomias*. In this section we follow the diagram about types of dysautonomia from a few pages ago.

> *Doctors can disagree about how to classify dysautonomias.*

As you read about the *dysautonomias,* keep in mind that the particular labels that are given for many of these conditions are "best guesses;" many labels refer to essentially the same set of symptoms; even with the same label, different people can have very different symptoms; and actual mechanisms for many of these conditions are not well understood. Further research will lead to discoveries about the causes of these conditions, and new, definitive names for the conditions.

> *The primary concern for the patient and doctor should be symptom management, which will provide relief and better quality of life.*

Changes in *autonomic nervous system* function can adversely affect health by **worsening another disease**. One example of this is the activation of the **sympathetic nervous system** during exercise in the cold, such as during shoveling snow. Both cold exposure and exercise increase activity of the *sympathetic nervous system.* Under normal circumstances this helps the person, by preserving and generating body heat and by delivering more blood to the muscles. The blood pressure and pulse rate increase, the work of the heart increases, and the blood flow to the heart muscle by the *coronary arteries* normally increases. But if the person has severe *coronary artery disease,* where the *coronary arteries* feeding the heart are narrowed, then when the work of the heart increases, due to activation of the *sympathetic nervous system,* the blood flow in the *coronary arteries* does not increase. This imbalance between the limited delivery of oxygen by the blood and the increased demand for oxygen can produce chest pain or pressure, heart attacks, or fatal abnormalities in heart rhythm. In other words, what would in other situations be a normal, helpful increase in *sympathetic nervous system* activity ends up worsening the health of the patient, in this case by turning "silent" *coronary artery disease* into a killer.

Changes in *autonomic nervous system* function can also be harmful, when activity of the system changes to **compensate** for abnormal functioning of a different body system. For instance, in *heart failure,* the heart fails to deliver an appropriate amount of blood to body organs. As compensation to improve the pump function of the heart, the *sympathetic nervous system* is activated. At the same time that this can improve the pump function of the heart, the activation of the *sympathetic nervous system* also increases the risk of fatal abnormal heart rhythms, increases the work of the heart, and promotes overgrowth of heart muscle, which can stiffen the heart walls and worsen the heart failure.

When doctors think about *dysautonomias,* they usually don't think about altered function of the *autonomic nervous system* worsening another disease, or about harmful effects of *compensatory activation* when another system fails. Instead, doctors think about abnormal function of the *autonomic nervous system* itself.

In general, there are four types of abnormal function of the *autonomic nervous system.* There may be acute overactivity, chronic overactivity, acute underactivity, and chronic underactivity. The next chapters describe these disorders.

In What Conditions is the Autonomic Nervous System Underactive?

Different parts of the autonomic nervous system are underactive in different disorders.

When the *parasympathetic nervous system* is underactive, the person has constipation, retention of urine in the bladder, a tendency to fast pulse rate, decreased salivation, and in men *impotence.* Several drugs can cause this combination of problems, but sometimes they result from failure of some part of the *parasympathetic nervous system.* Whether the problem is in the brain, in the nerve traffic from the brain, in the *ganglia* that act like transfer stations on the nervous system highway, in the nerve terminals preventing release of the chemical messenger, *acetylcholine,* or in the *receptors* for *acetylcholine* in the tissue, the effects in terms of the way the patient feels and looks are about the

> *Parasympathetic nervous system underactivity produces constipation, urinary problems, fast pulse rate, decreased spit, or (in men) an inability to have an erection.*

same. In other words, many different mechanisms can result in the same symptoms.

The *parasympathetic nervous system* is underactive in several types of *dysautonomia,* including *Parkinson's disease* with *autonomic failure, pure autonomic failure,* and *multiple system atrophy.* All these types of *dysautonomia* also feature underactivity of the *sympathetic nervous system* too, and they are discussed later in separate sections. Parasympathetic functions tend to decrease also with normal aging.

When the *sympathetic nervous system* is underactive, the person has a fall in blood pressure if the patient stands up, which is called *orthostatic hypotension.* Sympathetic failure produces a tendency to slow pulse rate and in men inability to ejaculate. Several drugs can cause this combination of problems, but sometimes they result from failure of some part of the *sympathetic nervous system.*

A fall in blood pressure when the patient stands (orthostatic hypotension) is an important sign of failure of the sympathetic nervous system.

As for underactivity of the *parasympathetic nervous system,* whether the problem is in the brain, in the nerve traffic from the brain, in the *ganglia,* in the nerve terminals preventing release of the chemical messenger, *norepinephrine,* or in the *receptors* for *norepinephrine* in the tissue, the effects in terms of the way the patient feels and looks are about the same.

Sweating and blood pressure are "automatic" functions controlled by different chemicals.

Since *acetylcholine* is the main chemical messenger used by the *sympathetic nervous system* for sweating, while *norepinephrine* is the main chemical messenger used by the *sympathetic nerve system* to tighten blood vessels and maintain blood pressure during standing, a patient with a specific problem in the production, release, or *receptors* for *norepinephrine* could have *orthostatic hypotension* and yet sweat normally.

The *sympathetic nervous system* is underactive in several types of *dysautonomia,* including *Parkinson's disease with autonomic failure, pure autonomic failure, and multiple system atrophy.* Acute *sympathetic failure* also appears to play a key role in fainting.

When the *adrenomedullary hormonal system* is underactive, the effects on the body are much more subtle than when the *parasympathetic nervous system* or the *sympathetic nervous system* is underactive. This is probably because the *adrenomedullary hormonal system* is activated in relatively unusual emergency situations. When you are at rest, your *adrenal glands* release very little *epinephrine* into the bloodstream.

Epinephrine (adrenaline) is one of the body's main hormones for regulating blood levels of *glucose,* one of the body's main fuels. Failure of the *adrenomedullary hormonal system* can cause a tendency to low glucose levels, a condition called *hypoglycemia.* This can be a major problem in patients who have *diabetes* and take injections of *insulin,* because failure of the *adrenomedullary hormonal system* in these patients can result in susceptibility to severe *hypoglycemia* reactions to the *insulin.*

Failure of the adrenomedullary hormonal system can cause a tendency to low glucose levels (hypoglycemia).

What is Orthostatic Hypotension?

Normally, when you stand up, you don't notice much that is different. Nevertheless, there are quite a few automatic, largely unconscious, reflexive changes directed by the brain that are required for tolerating the act of simply standing up. When the reflexes fail, the patient can't tolerate simply standing up. If the blood pressure falls by more than 20 millimeters of mercury between lying flat and standing up, this is called orthostatic hypotension.

Inability to tolerate standing up, or *orthostatic intolerance,* is a symptom, a complaint about something abnormal a person notices that provides subjective evidence of a disease. A fall in blood pressure when a person stands up, or *orthostatic hypotension,* is a sign, something a doctor can observe or measure that provides objective evidence of a disease. Neither *orthostatic intolerance* nor *orthostatic hypotension* is a diagnosis, which is a decision about the cause of a specific case of disease.

> *Orthostatic hypotension: a 20 point or larger fall in blood pressure when a person stands up from lying down.*

When a person stands up, this sets into motion an important reflex called the *baroreflex*. The *baroreflex* helps to maintain the blood pressure. When a person stands up, the force of gravity tends to pool blood in the legs and lower abdomen. This decreases the return of blood to the heart in the veins. The heart ejects less blood. *Baroreceptors* are tiny distortion receptors in the walls of large vessels and in the heart muscle. When the heart ejects less blood, information changes in nerves traveling from the *baroreceptors* to the brain. The brain responds by directing an increase in the activity of the *sympathetic nervous system*. The *sympathetic nerves* release *norepinephrine,* and the *norepinephrine* activates *receptors* on cells in the blood vessel walls. This tightens the blood vessels, and so the total resistance to blood flow in the body increases. In other words, the *total peripheral resistance increases.* Even though the total amount of blood ejected by the heart per minute *(cardiac output)* has decreased, the average *blood pressure* normally is maintained, due to the increase in *total peripheral resistance.*

You might understand the *baroreflex* better by thinking about the water pressure in a garden hose. The pressure is determined by how much the faucet is turned on and how much the nozzle is tightened. If you turned down the faucet, the pressure in the hose would decrease, and less water would come out the nozzle. If you wanted to keep the pressure in the hose the same, you could tighten the nozzle.

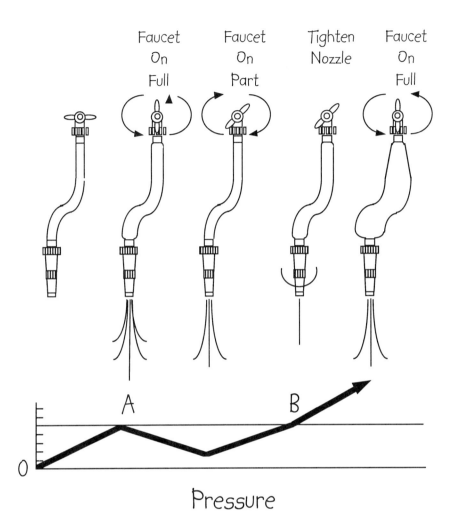

There are two ways to control the pressure in a garden hose: the faucet and the nozzle. There are two ways to control blood pressure: cardiac output and total peripheral resistance.

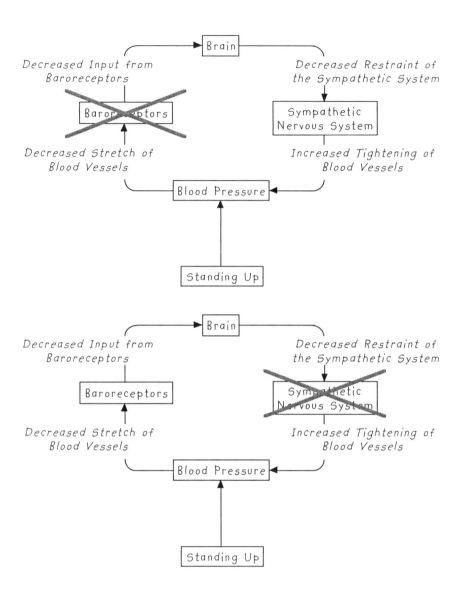

The baroreflex and sympathetic nervous system must both work, for a person to tolerate standing up.

Baroreflexes control the amount of tightening of the blood vessels. When a person stands up, the blood vessels tighten reflexively, helping maintain the blood pressure, and the main system responsible for tightening the vascular nozzle is the *sympathetic nervous system.* This explains why failure of the *sympathetic nervous system* always causes *orthostatic hypotension.*

> *In sympathetic nervous system failure, the patient can't tighten the "nozzle."*

Doctors may have different opinions about the amount of *orthostatic hypotension* that is clinically significant. Normally the systolic pressure falls slightly during standing up, because the heart is ejecting less blood, and normally the diastolic pressure does not fall at all, because of the reflexive constriction of blood vessels in the body as a whole. In general, if the *systolic blood pressure* (the peak pressure when the heart beats) decreases by more than 20 millimeters of mercury and the diastolic pressure decreases by more than 5 millimeters of mercury, then the patient has *orthostatic hypotension.*

Orthostatic hypotension is a key sign of *sympathetic neurocirculatory failure.* Any of several diseases can produce *orthostatic hypotension* from *sympathetic neurocirculatory failure.*

Sympathetic Neurocirculatory Failure

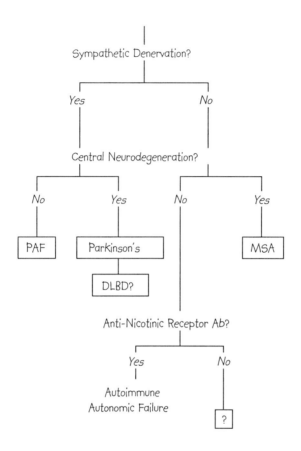

Sympathetic neurocirculatory failure has many potential causes.

These include *pure autonomic failure (PAF), multiple system atrophy (MSA), Parkinson's disease, diffuse Lewy body disease (DLBD), and autoimmune autonomic failure.* In these diseases, orthostatic hypotension occurs persistently and consistently.

There are other disorders where the patients cannot tolerate prolonged standing, even though they do not have persistent, consistent *orthostatic hypotension.* These *orthostatic intolerance* syndromes are discussed later.

Remember that neither *orthostatic intolerance* nor *orthostatic hypotension* is a disease. One is a symptom (or set of symptoms) that a person has when standing. The other is a sign that a doctor can measure.

Many factors besides *sympathetic neurocirculatory failure* can cause *orthostatic hypotension.* Prolonged bed rest for virtually any reason can do this. Indeed, in the American space program, a study of normal volunteers in perfect health found that after prolonged bed rest with the head slightly down, these healthy people often developed *orthostatic hypotension.* It should not be surprising that elderly, bedridden patients also routinely have *orthostatic hypotension. Orthostatic hypotension* can also result from conditions that cause depletion of blood volume, such as heavy menstrual periods or gastrointestinal hemorrhage from a bleeding ulcer.

There are many causes of orthostatic hypotension, besides sympathetic nervous system failure.

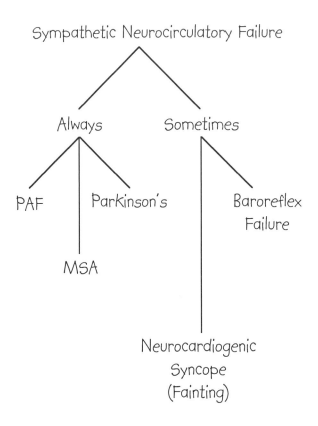

Sympathetic Neurocirculatory Failure

Always — Sometimes

PAF | Parkinson's — Baroreflex Failure

MSA

Neurocardiogenic Syncope (Fainting)

Failure of the sympathetic nervous system to regulate blood pressure occurs in both persistent diseases and occasional episodes.

What is Orthostatic Intolerance?

A major main way *dysautonomias* cause problems is by producing *orthostatic intolerance.* Remember that orthostatic intolerance is based on **symptoms**, such as dizziness or lightheadedness while standing. *Orthostatic intolerance* is not a **sign**, because it isn't something an observer can measure objectively. And it isn't a **disease** (although there are many diseases that produce *orthostatic intolerance*). The fact that there are many possible causes of *orthostatic intolerance* poses a challenge to any doctor trying to come up with a diagnosis to explain *orthostatic intolerance* in a particular patient.

Patients with orthostatic intolerance can't tolerate prolonged standing.

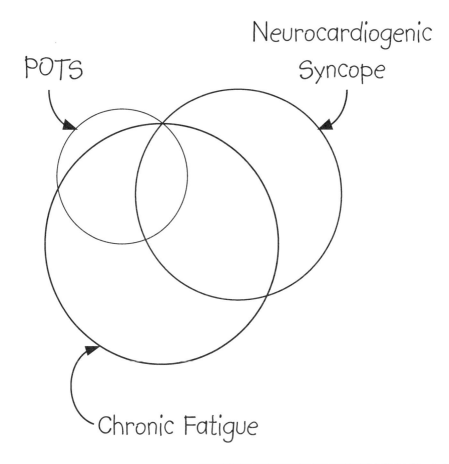

About 60% of patients with Chronic Fatigue Syndrome have Chronic Orthostatic Intolerance, with Postural Tachycardia Syndrome (POTS), Neurocardiogenic Syncope, or both.

Chronic Orthostatic Intolerance

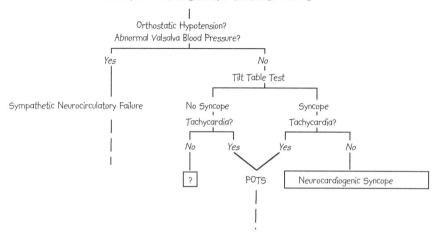

> *One approach in the diagnosis of chronic orthostatic intolerance is based on whether the patient has a fall in blood pressure during standing (orthostatic hypotension).*

Patients with *Chronic Fatigue Syndrome* often have *orthostatic intolerance.* The *orthostatic intolerance* can be associated with *postural tachycardia syndrome (POTS), neurocardiogenic syncope,* or both.

A starting point in identifying a cause of *orthostatic intolerance* is to determine whether the patient has failure of the *sympathetic nervous system* to regulate the heart and blood vessels correctly. We call this *sympathetic neurocirculatory failure.* In *dysautonomias* that produce

Chronic Orthostatic Intolerance

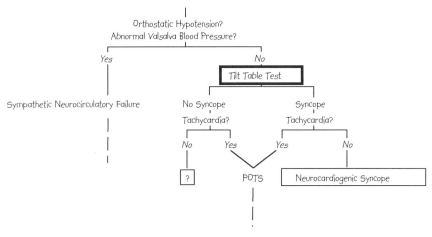

Doctors often do tilt table testing in patients who cannot tolerate standing (orthostatic intolerance) and do not have a fall in blood pressure during standing (orthostatic hypotension).

---

chronic sympathetic neurocirculatory failure, the patient always has a fall in blood pressure during standing, or *orthostatic hypotension.*

In other forms of *chronic orthostatic intolerance,* the person does not have *sympathetic neurocirculatory failure,* and the blood pressure does not fall consistently when the person stands up (although the person can have delayed *orthostatic hypotension* after many minutes of standing). Instead, the person feels dizzy or lightheaded during standing, even while the blood pressure is maintained. *Orthostatic hypotension* can produce *orthostatic intolerance,* but *orthostatic intolerance* can occur without *orthostatic hypotension.*

In the evaluation of a patient with *chronic orthostatic intolerance,* where the patient does not have evidence of *sympathetic neurocirculatory failure,* doctors often prescribe a *tilt table test.* The chapter about testing for *dysautonomias* discusses the *tilt table test.* In general, there are two types of positive *tilt table test* result. If the patient has an excessive, progressively more severe increase in pulse rate during the tilting, then this would be consistent with *postural tachycardia syndrome,* or *POTS.* If the patient has a decrease in the level of consciousness and finally loses consciousness *(syncope),* then this would be consistent with *neurocardiogenic syncope.* The loss of consciousness is virtually always associated with a fall in blood pressure, or *neurally mediated hypotension.* A tilt table test can also yield results consistent with both *POTS* and *neurocardiogenic syncope,* such as when the patient has a large increase in pulse rate, followed by a sudden fall in pulse rate back to normal, *neurally mediated hypotension,* and *syncope.*

Once a diagnosis of *POTS* is made, the workup may continue, to determine if the rapid pulse is part of a primary problem or is part of a compensation. The section about *POTS* discusses this workup.

In patients with *neurocardiogenic syncope,* the *sympathetic nervous system* can fail to work correctly only once in a while, in episodes, and in these episodes a person can feel faint or actually lose consciousness. A common form of *dysautonomia* where the *sympathetic nervous system* fails episodically is in *fainting,* which also has been called *neurally mediated syncope, neurocardiogenic syncope,* or the *common faint.* It is important to recognize that between episodes of fainting, patients with repeated episodes of *neurocardiogenic syncope* often do not feel well. In fact, they can complain of the same non-specific symptoms that patients with *POTS* describe, such as fatigue, heat intolerance, headache, exercise intolerance, and *orthostatic intolerance.*

> *The sympathetic nervous system fails when people faint.*

Much less commonly, *orthostatic intolerance* reflects failure of the *baroreflex.* In this situation, the *sympathetic nervous system* is not activated appropriately in response to a decrease in blood pressure or in response to a decrease in *venous return* to the heart. Seemingly paradoxically, *baroreflex failure* does not necessarily cause *orthostatic hypotension,* but it does always cause large swings in blood pressure, both high and low, because of the inability of the *baroreflex* to keep the blood pressure within limits.

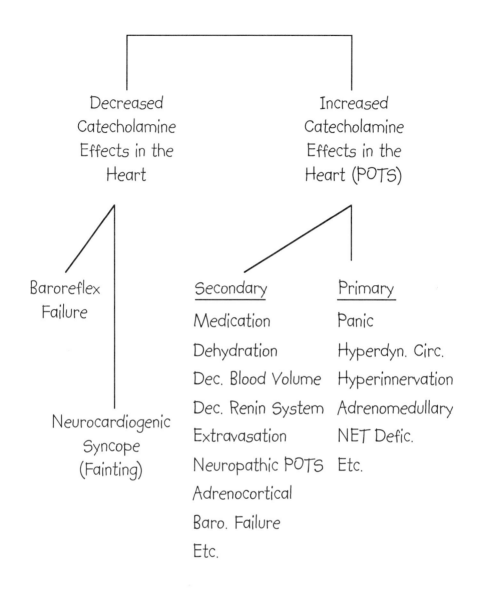

Decreased Catecholamine Effects in the Heart

Increased Catecholamine Effects in the Heart (POTS)

Baroreflex Failure

Neurocardiogenic Syncope (Fainting)

<u>Secondary</u>

Medication

Dehydration

Dec. Blood Volume

Dec. Renin System

Extravasation

Neuropathic POTS

Adrenocortical

Baro. Failure

Etc.

<u>Primary</u>

Panic

Hyperdyn. Circ.

Hyperinnervation

Adrenomedullary

NET Defic.

Etc.

Orthostatic intolerance can be associated with increased or decreased effects of adrenaline-like chemicals in the heart.

Pure Autonomic Failure

This and the following sections describe several specific *dysautonomias*. The description is not meant to be exhaustive, and individual patients can have symptoms or signs that overlap.

Pure Autonomic Failure (PAF)

- *Mid-aged or elderly of either sex and any race*
- *Chronic, persistent fall in blood pressure during standing up*
- *No signs of brain disease*
- *Not inherited or infectious*
- *Can go one for many years*

Pure autonomic failure (PAF) features persistent falls in blood pressure when the patient stands—orthostatic hypotension—in the absence of signs of central nervous system disease and in the absence of other known causes of orthostatic hypotension. The *orthostatic hypotension* results from *sympathetic neurocirculatory failure*.

Pure autonomic failure, while chronic and causing disability, is not thought to be lethal.

Patients report progressively worsening dizziness standing up or after a large meal. Often they have decreased sweating. Because of severe *orthostatic hypotension, pure autonomic failure* patients often learn to sit or stand with their legs twisted pretzel-like, since this decreases pooling of blood in the legs. In men, impotence can be an early symptom.

In *patients with pure autonomic failure, blood pressure* responses to the *Valsalva maneuver* show the abnormal pattern that indicates *sympathetic neurocirculatory failure.* The *Valsalva maneuver* is discussed in the chapter about tests for *dysautonomias.*

The *sympathetic neurocirculatory failure* and *orthostatic hypotension* in pure autonomic failure typically result from loss of *sympathetic nerve terminals.*

Drug tests can confirm a diagnosis of *pure autonomic failure.* Because of the loss of *sympathetic nerve terminals,* drugs that release *norepinephrine* from *sympathetic nerves,* such as *yohimbine, amphetamine,* and *ephedrine,* produce relatively small increases in *blood pressure.* In contrast, drugs that directly stimulate *norepinephrine* receptors, such as *midodrine* and *phenylephrine* (Neo-Synephrine™) constrict blood vessels and increase *blood pressure.*

Because of the phenomenon of *"denervation supersensitivity,"* where *receptors* for *norepinephrine* increase and other adaptive processes probably occur that exaggerate constriction of blood vessels, patients with *pure autonomic failure* can have surprisingly large increases in blood pressure in response to the receptor-stimulating drugs.

As a result of loss of sympathetic nerve terminals, plasma *norepinephrine* levels typically are low in *PAF,* even with the patient lying down, and the levels fail to increase when the patient stands. In response to the above drugs, *plasma norepinephrine levels* fail to change as much as expected.

Another way to identify *PAF* is from *sympathetic neuroimaging.* In this type of test, the patient receives an injection of a radioactive drug that gets taken up by *sympathetic nerve terminals.* The *sympathetic nerves* in organs such as the heart become radioactive, and the nerves can be visualized by scans that detect where the radioactivity is, in a manner similar to commonly used clinical tests such as bone scans or brain scans. Since in *PAF* the *sympathetic nerve terminals* usually are absent in the organs, scanning after injection of one of these drugs fails to visualize the sympathetic *innervation.* *Sympathetic neuroimaging* tests such as *fluorodopamine PET* scanning of the chest usually produce remarkably graphic results in *PAF,* with a failure to visualize the heart walls at all.

No one knows what causes *pure autonomic failure.* It is not inherited, and no known environmental toxin causes it.

Treatment of *pure autonomic failure* is directed mainly at the *orthostatic hypotension,* which virtually always is severe and disabling. *Fludrocortisone,* a high salt diet, and *potassium* supplementation are the mainstays of treatment. Clinicians usually recommend elevation of the head of the bed. Body stockings may or may not help. The patient should not take large meals, because this may cause the *blood pressure* to decrease. Drugs that release *norepinephrine* from *sympathetic nerves,* such as *ephedrine, Ritalin™,* or *yohimbine,* may not work, because of the lack of nerve terminals, whereas drugs that artificially stimulate *receptors* for *norepinephrine,* such as *midodrine,* can be very effective.

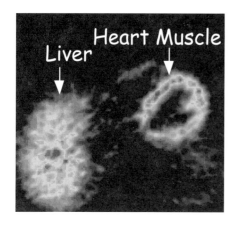

Blood Flow
PET Scan

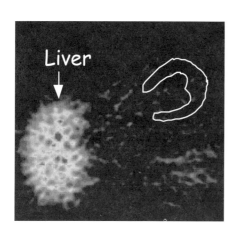

Sympathetic Nerve
PET Scan

Patients with Pure Autonomic Failure typically have a loss of sympathetic nerves in the heart muscle.

Multiple System Atrophy

Multiple system atrophy ("MSA") is a disease that involves progressive degeneration of multiple portions of the nervous system, including portions that regulate the *autonomic nervous system.* Several unconscious "vegetative" functions fail, such as digestion, urination, speech and swallowing mechanisms, and cardiovascular reflexes. Unlike *pure autonomic failure, MSA* is unfortunately a disease that is progressive and eventually lethal. On average, patients survive for about a half dozen years after the diagnosis is made. *MSA* differs from *multiple sclerosis,* which is characterized clinically by remissions and exacerbations and by relatively few changes in functions of the *autonomic nervous system.*

Multiple System Atrophy (MSA)
- *Mid-aged or elderly of either sex and any race*
- *Not inherited or infectious*
- *Chronic, persistent autonomic failure*
- *Signs of brain disease, such as slurred speech, rigidity, tremor, poor coordination*
- *Relentless progression over years*

No one knows what causes *MSA*. It is not inherited, and no known environmental toxin causes it. According to one view, *MSA* results from a form of *auto-immune* process, where the patient's immune system attacks and destroys particular brain cells.

MSA has different forms, which result in somewhat different symptoms and signs. In the *parkinsonian* form of *MSA (MSAp)* the patient has symptoms and signs of *Parkinson's disease,* such as shakiness of the hands *(tremor)* that is most prominent at rest and decreases with intentional movements, muscular rigidity, and slow initiation of movement. Unlike in Parkinson's disease, these problems usually do not respond well to treatment with Sinemet™, the most commonly used drug for Parkinson's disease.

In the *cerebellar* form of *MSA (MSA$_C$)* the patient has symptoms and signs of failure of the *cerebellum,* which is a part of the brain that plays an important role in coordinated movements, coherent speech, balance, and accurate gait. If the patient has a *tremor,* it worsens with intentional movements. The typical patient also has slurred speech and a wide-based, "drunken sailor" type gait.

In the *mixed* form of *MSA (MSA$_M$)* the patient has a mixture of *parkinsonian* and *cerebellar* symptoms and signs.

MSA always involves one or more symptoms or signs of failure of the *autonomic nervous system.* Failure of the *parasympathetic nervous system* produces *urinary retention* and *incontinence, constipation, erectile impotence,* and *decreased salivation.* Failure of the *sympathetic nervous system* produces a fall in *blood pressure* when the patient stands up *(orthostatic hypotension)* or after a meal *(post-prandial hypotension),* resulting in symptoms such as dizziness, weakness, or faintness upon standing or after eating.

MSA with failure of sympathetic reflexes *(sympathetic neurocirculatory failure)* is also known as the *Shy-Drager syndrome.* The most clear sign of *sympathetic neurocirculatory failure* is *orthostatic hypotension.*

MSA with a fall in blood pressure standing is also called the Shy-Drager syndrome.

Some investigators have equated *MSA* with the *Shy-Drager syndrome.* Others have considered *MSA* as an umbrella diagnosis that includes the *Shy-Drager syndrome* when *orthostatic hypotension* figures prominently in the clinical presentation but also includes forms where signs of *cerebellar atrophy* or of *Parkinson's disease* stand out. A recent proposal has recommended discarding using the *Shy-Drager syndrome* as a diagnosis.

Based on clinical findings and results of *autonomic function testing,* we have proposed a somewhat different classification scheme that distinguishes *MSA* with predominantly *parasympathetic* or other *brainstem degeneration* from *MSA* with predominantly *sympathetic* degeneration, so that the *Shy-Drager syndrome* is synonymous with *MSA* and *sympathetic neurocirculatory failure.*

Symptoms and signs of *parasympathetic* degeneration include constipation and decreased urinary bladder tone, resulting in urinary incontinence, frequency, urgency, and the need for self-catheterization. Symptoms and signs of other brainstem degeneration include particular abnormalities in eye movements *("progressive supranuclear palsy"),* slurred speech, dyscoordinated swallowing, abnormal breathing, and repeated *aspiration,* where swallowed food goes into the airway. These problems can occur in patients with *MSA* who do not have *orthostatic hypotension* or other evidence of failure of the *sympathetic nervous system.*

In *MSA,* it is thought that the *autonomic failure* reflects loss of the ability to regulate *sympathetic* and *parasympathetic nerve traffic* to the *nerve terminals,* but the terminals themselves are intact. This appears to be a major difference between *MSA* and the usual form of *pure autonomic failure,* where the *autonomic failure* includes a loss of *sympathetic nerve terminals.* Because of the presence of intact *sympathetic nerve terminals,* patients with *MSA* have increases in blood pressure when they receive drugs such as *yohimbine* that release *norepinephrine* from sympathetic nerve terminals and have decreases in blood pressure when they receive drugs such as *trimethaphan* that decrease release of *norepinephrine* from *sympathetic nerve terminals.*

The fact that *trimethaphan,* which works by blocking transmission of autonomic nerve impulses in the *ganglia,* decreases blood pressure in patients with *MSA* means that in *MSA* the problem is not so much decreased *autonomic nerve traffic* as failure of the brain to regulate that traffic appropriately.

The widely used dietary supplement or herbal remedy, *ma huang,* is *ephedrine,* which releases *norepinephrine* from *sympathetic nerve terminals.* Since patients with *MSA and sympathetic neurocirculatory failure* have intact *sympathetic nerve terminals,* and they also have failure of the brain to regulate *sympathetic nerve traffic* appropriately via *baroreflexes,* taking *ma huang* can evoke a dangerous increase in blood pressure in these patients.

Patients with *MSA* appear to have approximately normal *sympathetic nerve traffic* to intact *sympathetic nerve terminals* when they are lying down, and so while they are lying down they usually have normal *plasma* levels *norepinephrine*, the chemical messenger of the *sympathetic nervous system.* The patients often have a failure to increase *sympathetic nerve traffic* when they stand up, and so they have a failure to increase plasma *norepinephrine* levels normally when they stand up. In contrast, patients with *pure autonomic failure,* who have a loss of *sympathetic nerve terminals,* usually have low plasma *norepinephrine* levels even when they are lying down.

Another way to distinguish *MSA* from *pure autonomic failure* is from *sympathetic neuroimaging*. In this type of test, the patient receives an injection of a radioactive drug that gets taken up by *sympathetic nerve terminals*. The *sympathetic nerves* in organs such as the heart become radioactive, and the nerves can be visualized by scans that detect where the radioactivity is, in a manner similar to commonly used clinical tests such as bone scans or brain scans. Since in *MSA* the *sympathetic nerve terminals* are present in the organs, scanning after injection of one of these drugs visualizes the sympathetic *innervation*. In contrast, in *pure autonomic failure* (and in *Parkinson's disease,* discussed elsewhere), where the *sympathetic nerve terminals* typically are lost, *sympathetic neuroimaging* fails to visualize the sympathetic *innervation* of the heart.

The parkinsonian form of MSA can be difficult to distinguish from Parkinson's disease.

Distinguishing the *parkinsonian* form of *MSA* (*MSAp*) from *Parkinson's disease* with *autonomic failure* can be a difficult diagnostic challenge. As mentioned above, one way to distinguish these diseases is from *sympathetic neuroimaging,* since patients with *MSA* have normal sympathetic *innervation* of the heart, and patients with

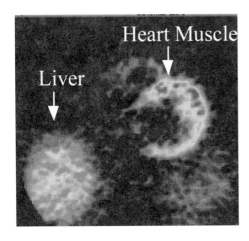

Blood Flow
PET Scan

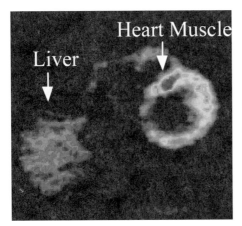

Sympathetic Nerve
PET Scan (Normal)

MSA patients have normal sympathetic nerves in the heart muscle.

Parkinson's disease and orthostatic hypotension have a loss of sympathetic *innervation* of the heart.

Treatment of *MSA* is directed at the symptoms and signs, such as *orthostatic hypotension,* and does not prevent or delay the progressive deterioration of the nervous system.

Because of steadily worsening difficulty with coordination of speech and swallowing mechanisms, patients with MSA have a high risk of *aspiration,* aspiration pneumonia, bloodstream infection, or sudden death from stopped breathing.

Parkinson's Disease with Orthostatic Hypotension

Orthostatic hypotension, a fall in blood pressure when the patient stands up, occurs fairly commonly in *Parkinson's disease.* Neurologists have presumed that the *orthostatic hypotension* results from treatment with *levodopa,* or else the patient doesn't really have *Parkinson's disease* but has a different disease, such as *"striatonigral degeneration"* or *multiple system atrophy.*

Parkinson's Disease with Orthostatic Hypotension

- *Elderly of either sex and any race*
- *Signs of Parkinson's disease, such as slow movements, rigidity, tremor*
- *Movement problem improves with Sinemet™ (DOPA+carbidopa)*
- *Chronic, persistent fall in blood pressure standing*
- *Can be inherited*
- *Slow progression over years*

Evidence is accumulating that all patients with *Parkinson's disease* and *orthostatic hypotension*—even patients off *levodopa* or never treated with *levodopa*—have failure of regulation of the heart and blood vessels by the *sympathetic nervous system*. In other words, in *Parkinson's disease, orthostatic hypotension* reflects *sympathetic neurocirculatory failure* and is therefore a form of *dysautonomia*.

Patients with Parkinson's disease and a fall in blood pressure when they stand up have a form of dysautonomia.

In patients with *Parkinson's disease* and *orthostatic hypotension*, the *sympathetic neurocirculatory failure* appears to result from loss of *sympathetic nerve terminals* in the body as a whole. Because of the *sympathetic denervation,* there is a decreased amount of *norepinephrine* available for release in response to standing up, and failure to release an adequate amount of *norepinephrine* explains the *orthostatic hypotension* in *Parkinson's disease.*

Many patients with Parkinson's disease who do not have a fall in blood pressure when they stand up still have a loss of sympathetic nerves in the heart.

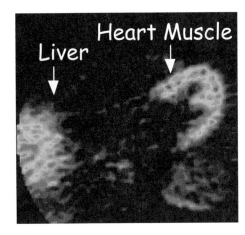

Blood Flow
PET Scan

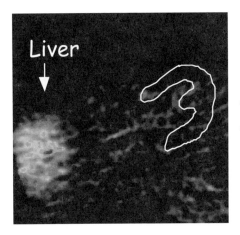

Sympathetic Nerve
PET Scan

Patients with Parkinson's disease often have
a loss of sympathetic nerves in the heart
muscle.

Surprisingly, most patients with *Parkinson's disease* who
do not have *orthostatic hypotension* nevertheless have

neuroimaging evidence for a loss of *sympathetic nerve supply* in the heart. *Parkinson's disease* therefore appears to be not only a disease of control of movement but also is *a dysautonomia,* because of the loss of *sympathetic nerve terminals.*

Pure autonomic failure also features *orthostatic hypotension* from loss of *sympathetic nerve terminals.* Some elderly patients with *pure autonomic failure* have subtle signs of *parkinsonism,* such as a mask-like facial expression and a type of stiffness of muscles. *Pure autonomic failure* can be difficult to distinguish from early or mild *Parkinson's disease* in these patients.

The long-term outlook in *Parkinson's disease* with *orthostatic hypotension* from *sympathetic neurocirculatory failure* seems about the same as in Parkinson's disease without *orthostatic hypotension.* The *orthostatic hypotension* does not appear to worsen with *levodopa* treatment, although the blood pressure both while lying down and when standing up can decrease.

The functional significance of loss of *sympathetic innervation* of the heart in *Parkinson's disease* remains unknown. One would presume that this would cause or contribute to an inability to tolerate exercise.

Treatments used for *Parkinson's disease* with *orthostatic hypotension* from *sympathetic neurocirculatory failure* include Florinef™ and a high salt diet, midodrine, frequent small meals and avoidance of large meals, and elevation of the head of the bed on blocks at night.

Treatments that depend on release of *norepinephrine* from *sympathetic nerve terminals,* such as *ephedrine, d-amphetamine, methylphenidate,* and *yohimbine,* may not work, because of the loss of the nerve terminals.

Patients with Parkinson's disease also often complain of constipation and urinary retention, urgency, and incontinence. These might reflect a form of failure of the parasympathetic nervous system; however, whether this is the case remains poorly understood. Failure of the parasympathetic nervous system supply to the heart appears to cause the constant pulse rate seen in most patients with Parkinson's disease and orthostatic hypotension; however, whether this reflects a loss of parasympathetic nerve terminals or a problem in regulating parasympathetic nerve traffic to intact terminals remains unknown.

Postural Tachycardia Syndrome (POTS)

Patients with the *postural tachycardia syndrome (postural orthostatic tachycardia syndrome, POTS)* have an excessive increase in pulse rate during standing.

> *POTS patients have too rapid a pulse rate when they stand, and usually several other non-specific problems.*

That being said, it should be pointed out at the beginning of this discussion that different research groups have different views about the classification of *dysautonomias,* and especially about *POTS* and *chronic orthostatic intolerance.* Just having a fast pulse rate while standing would not necessarily be harmful and cannot be a *syndrome,* which always involves more than a single symptom or sign.

POTS is associated with a variety of other symptoms that, when thought of individually, are not specific for any particular disease process. These include inability to tolerate prolonged standing, a tendency to faint, chest pain, cool, sweaty extremities, migraine-like headache, pain in the back of the neck or shoulders, heat

Postural Tachycardia Syndrome

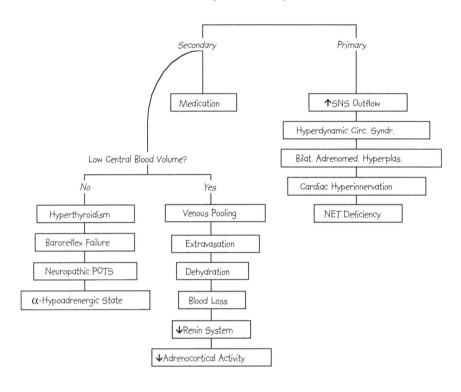

POTS has many potential causes.

---

intolerance, chronic fatigue, exercise intolerance, shortness of breath on exertion, and panic/anxiety. At least some of these symptoms are thought to reflect increased effects of the *catecholamines, norepinephrine (noradrenaline)* or *epinephrine (adrenaline),* in the heart, from overactivity of the *sympathetic nervous system* or *adrenomedullary hormonal system,* or both.

Most cases occur in relatively young (14-45 years old) women (female:male ratio about 5:1).

Postural Tachycardia Syndrome (POTS)
- *Mainly young adult women*
- *Too rapid pulse rate during standing*
- *Several non-specific associated problems (inability to tolerate prolonged standing, fatigue, faintness, chest pain, heart "flip-flops," heat intolerance, exercise intolerance, tendency to panic)*
- *Variable outlook, can improve*
- *Not life-threatening*

Some investigators view *POTS* as synonymous with *chronic orthostatic intolerance.* As discussed later, the condition has features also suggestive of *hyperdynamic circulation syndrome* or "*neurasthenia.*" The many terms that have been used probably reflect different emphases by different research groups and large gaps in knowledge about the underlying mechanisms in individual patients.

The *orthostatic tachycardia* usually occurs without *orthostatic hypotension.* The finding of *orthostatic hypotension* does not exclude a diagnosis of POTS, however, and *delayed orthostatic hypotension* can occur in this condition.

> *POTS is a syndrome, not a single disease, and can have any of several causes.*

Most *postural tachycardia* is secondary to identifiable problems, such as side effects of medications or dehydration from chronic illness. When the cause is not readily identified, and the patient has other complaints discussed below, then the patient is thought to have *postural tachycardia syndrome,* or *POTS.*

The occurrence of a rapid pulse rate when a person stands is necessary but is not sufficient to diagnose *POTS.* The key word in *postural tachycardia syndrome* is the word, *"syndrome."* A *syndrome* is a set of symptoms that occur together. Patients with *POTS* not only have a rapid pulse rate when they stand up, they also have several other symptoms, such as *orthostatic intolerance,* chronic fatigue, heat intolerance, exercise intolerance, headache, chest pain, palpitations, neuropsychological complaints such as disturbed sleep, anxiety, or depression, and disability.

Trying to identify a specific cause in a particular patient with *POTS* can be a great challenge to clinicians. There are probably as many causes of a fast pulse rate as there are of a fever, and all the symptoms of *POTS* are not specific for any single disease.

Researchers have thought that usually in *POTS,* *sympathetic nerve* traffic to the heart is increased as a compensation. The compensation could be for a decrease in the amount of blood returning to the heart or a decrease in the *total peripheral resistance* to blood flow when the patient stands up. Either situation could alter information from the *baroreceptors* to the brain, leading to a reflexive increase in *sympathetic nervous system* activity directed by the brain.

Low Blood Volume

There are many causes for a decrease in the amount of blood returning to the heart when a patient is standing. The possibility of *blood volume* depletion or excessive pooling of blood in the legs during standing up has drawn particular attention. Indeed, low *blood volume* was noted in the first case report of *POTS,* and the response, at least in the short run, to infused *normal saline* can be dramatic.

Low *blood volume* in turn can result from blood loss, from failure of the bone marrow to make an adequate number of red blood cells, or from failure of hormone systems such as the *renin-angiotensin-aldosterone* system. In addition, blood volume can fall while a person stands, due to leakage of fluid out of the blood vessels into the tissues *(extravasation).* Finally, an "effective" low blood volume can occur, when the blood pools excessively in the veins after a person stands, such as because of a lack of muscular "tone" in the vein walls.

Delayed orthostatic hypotension in *POTS* is also thought to result from a progressive, exaggerated decline in *blood volume* during prolonged standing, from leakage of fluid into the tissues through blood vessel walls *(extravasation)*. Consistent with excessive blood pooling in the legs or lower abdomen during *orthostasis*, inflation of a *military antishock trousers (MAST) suit* reduces substantially the increase in heart rate in response to *orthostasis* in patients with *POTS*.

Neuropathic POTS

In *partial dysautonomia,* or *neuropathic POTS,* there is thought to be a patchy loss of sympathetic *innervation,* such as in the legs. When the patient stands up, the blood pools in the veins of the legs, and less blood returns to the heart, or else the arterioles fail to constrict, and the total resistance to blood flow decreases. In response to either or both of these abnormalities, the *sympathetic nervous system* supply to the heart would be stimulated reflexively.

There are other possible causes of decreased *total peripheral resistance* that might reflexively increase *sympathetic nervous system* traffic to the heart. For instance, any of several drugs block *receptors* for *norepinephrine* in blood vessel walls, and other drugs directly relax blood vessel walls.

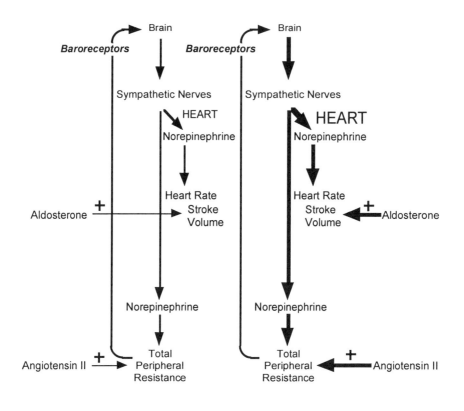

NORMAL   DEHYDRATION
or
BLOOD LOSS

> *Dehydration, blood loss, or other causes of decreased blood volume can produce a condition that looks like POTS.*

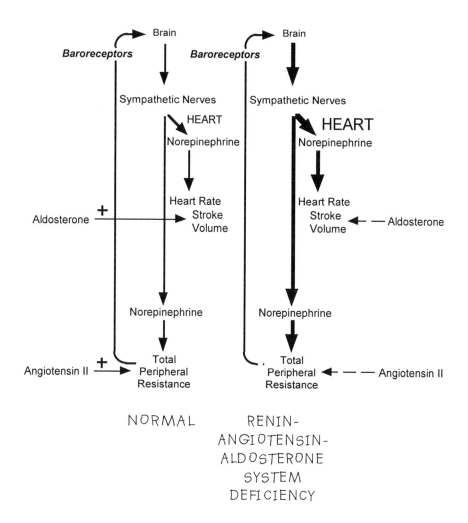

NORMAL   RENIN-
ANGIOTENSIN-
ALDOSTERONE
SYSTEM
DEFICIENCY

POTS can result from failure of a key system regulating salt balance and blood volume in the body, called the renin-angiotensin-aldosterone system.

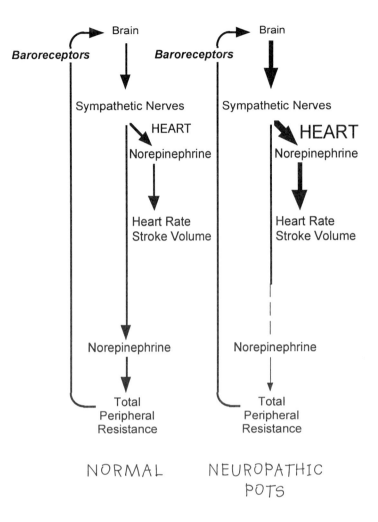

NORMAL   NEUROPATHIC POTS

In "neuropathic POTS," sympathetic nerves to the heart are thought to be overactive, as a compensation for loss of sympathetic nerves elsewhere.

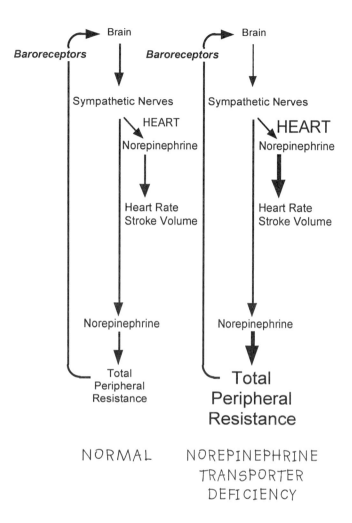

NORMAL

NOREPINEPHRINE
TRANSPORTER
DEFICIENCY

Rarely, POTS can result from failure to inactivate norepinephrine, a key chemical messenger of nerves in the heart.

In rare patients, POTS results from deficiency of the *cell membrane norepinephrine transporter,* or *NET.*

Hyperadrenergic Orthostatic Intolerance

In *hyperadrenergic orthostatic intolerance*, the problem is thought to be a **primary** abnormality in the functioning or regulation of the *autonomic nervous system* itself.

For instance, in *acute baroreflex failure,* the brain does not respond appropriately to information from the cardiovascular system, and the *sympathetic nervous system* is activated inappropriately. In *acute baroreflex failure, orthostatic intolerance* is associated with large swings in blood pressure, because of the inability of the *baroreflexes* to keep the blood pressure in check, with episodes of extreme high blood pressure and fast pulse rate. Because of this failure, relatively minor stimuli can produce large increases in the activity of the *sympathetic nervous system.*

Another cause of *hyperadrenergic orthostatic intolerance* is decreased function of the *cell membrane norepinephrine transporter,* also called *NET deficiency.* The *cell membrane norepinephrine transporter* plays a key role in inactivating *norepinephrine.* Normally, most of the *norepinephrine* released from *sympathetic nerve terminals* is "recycled," by being taken back up into the nerve terminals. When the *transporter* is underactive, more *norepinephrine* is delivered to its *receptors* in the heart and blood vessel walls for a given amount of *norepinephrine release,* producing an exaggerated increase in pulse rate and blood pressure in situations where the *sympathetic nervous system* is activated.

In a related syndrome, called the *hyperdynamic circulation syndrome,* the patients have a fast pulse rate all the time, variable high blood pressure, increased heart rate responses to the drug, *isoproterenol*, and increased plasma *norepinephrine* and *epinephrine* levels at rest and during provocative maneuvers. *ß-Adrenoceptor blockers* such as *Inderal*™ or *benzodiazepines* such as *Valium*™ improve the syndrome. It is unclear whether patients with this syndrome have an increased frequency of later development of established *hypertension.* Episodes of fast pulse rate and increased blood pressure can be associated with blotchy flushing of the face, neck, and upper chest.

"Neurasthenia" a term introduced in the late 1860s. refers to a syndrome initially described in Civil War soldiers. Also called *neurocirculatory asthenia,* the syndrome consists of a large number of symptoms, including breathlessness, *palpitations,* chest pain, dizziness, shortness of breath on exertion, fatigue, excessive sweating, trembling, flushing, dry mouth, numbness and tingling feelings, irritability, and exercise intolerance.

Most modern research about *neurocirculatory asthenia* has been conducted in Russia. Western cardiovascular researchers rarely use this term. The symptoms resemble those in *POTS,* and as in *POTS,* the multiplicity of symptoms contrasts with a relative lack of signs, which all are non-specific—relatively fast pulse rate, relatively rapid breathing, facial and neck flushing, slight *tremor,* sweaty palms, a "functional" heart murmur, and hyperactive kneejerk reflexes, with generally normal resting blood pressure. Just as in *POTS* or the *hyperdynamic circulation syndrome,* in *neurasthenia* injections of *adrenaline* can evoke these symptoms. *ß-Adrenoceptor blockers* often normalize the cardiovascular findings without affecting the other symptoms and signs. Drugs such as *caffeine* can evoke fast pulse rate, increased ventilation, tremor, and sweatiness in patients with *neurocirculatory asthenia.*

In another related condition, *inappropriate sinus tachycardia,* the heart rate is increased to 100 beats per minute or more, even under resting conditions. *Radiofrequency ablation* of the *sinus node,* the heart's pacemaker area, is considered for patients with *inappropriate sinus tachycardia* who are resistant to treatment with medications.

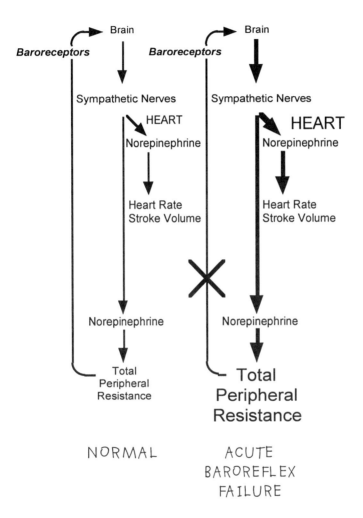

NORMAL

ACUTE
BAROREFLEX
FAILURE

Failure of the baroreflex can produce a condition that looks like POTS.

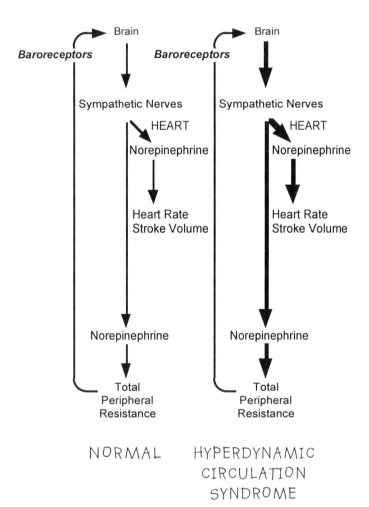

NORMAL   HYPERDYNAMIC
CIRCULATION
SYNDROME

The hyperdynamic circulation syndrome can cause POTS.

As discussed below, the *POTS* syndromes differ from *neurocardiogenic syncope (neurally mediated syncope),* in that patients with *neurocardiogenic syncope* have inhibition, rather than stimulation, of the *sympathetic nervous system,* at least during acute episodes. Patients with *POTS* often have increased plasma levels of *norepinephrine,* the chemical messenger of the sympathetic nervous system, especially when they are standing up. Indeed, according to one suggestion, criteria for diagnosing *chronic orthostatic intolerance* include an upright plasma *norepinephrine* level of 600 pg/ml or more; however, whether increased sympathetic outflow constitutes a primary abnormality or compensatory response usually is unknown in an individual patient.

In general, one would predict that if the *orthostatic tachycardia* were primary, then treating it would help the patient, but if the *orthostatic tachycardia* were secondary, then treating the problem would not help the patient. Keeping this principle in mind can help to understand how one patient may feel better from treatment with a beta-blocker, which forces the pulse rate to go down, while another may not feel better at all, even though the pulse rate has decreased to the same extent.

> *Treatment of POTS should be tailored to the individual patient.*

The first step in management of *chronic orthostatic intolerance* is to search carefully for common, reversible causes, such as *diabetes*, weight loss, prolonged bed rest, debilitating diseases, and medications.

Medical treatments for *POTS* generally have attempted to increase *blood volume,* such as using Florinef™ and liberal salt and water intake, injections of *erythropoietin,* or infusions of saline intravenously; block fast pulse rates, such as using *ß-adrenoceptor blockers* or *sinus node ablation;* decrease exaggerated *norepinephrine* release, such as using *clonidine, α-methylDOPA,* or *moxonidine;* or enhance *vasoconstriction*, such as using *midodrine, ergotamine,* or *octreotide.* Other treatments include venous compression hose, calf muscle resistance training, exercise training, or even insertion of a pacemaker.

Often these treatments, while helpful, do not bring the patients back to a sense of normal health. Over the course of months or even years, the patients can improve, or else they learn to cope with a chronic, debilitating, but not life-threatening disorder.

Neurocardiogenic Syncope

Syncope is sudden loss of consciousness associated with loss of muscle tone and the regaining of consciousness within a few minutes.

> *Syncope is sudden loss of consciousness (you black out) that is associated with loss of muscle tone (you go limp) and reverses rapidly (you wake up within minutes.)*

Neurocardiogenic syncope, which is also called *vasovagal syncope, vasodepressor syncope, neurally mediated syncope,* and the *common faint,* is by far the most common cause of sudden loss of consciousness in the general population.

In *neurocardiogenic presyncope,* the patient feels like he or she will faint but does not actually lose consciousness.

Most patients with frequent episodes of *neurocardiogenic syncope* recognize early signs of fainting coming on and are usually able to abort the episode before *syncope* actually occurs.

Neurocardiogenic syncope is most common in young adult women and in children.

> *Neurocardiogenic syncope is fainting. Neurocardiogenic presyncope is near-fainting but without actual loss of consciousness.*

In mid-aged or elderly adults, *syncope* is more likely to be a sign of a heart problem (abnormal heart rhythm, abnormal conduction of electrical impulses in the heart, or heart valve problem) or *orthostatic hypotension.* In patients where neurocardiogenic syncope is a frequent problem, even between episodes the patients often feel unwell, with an inability to tolerate prolonged standing, chronic fatigue, headache, and chest pain.

Neurocardiogenic syncope can resemble *POTS.* Both disorders mainly involve young adult women, (although in children *neurocardiogenic syncope* may be more common than *POTS),* and both are associated with inability to tolerate prolonged standing, chronic fatigue, headache, and chest pain (although *POTS* may more commonly involve symptoms about multiple body systems). In both conditions the patients have a tendency to near-fainting or fainting spells, especially while standing. *Neurocardiogenic syncope* does appear to differ from *POTS,* in that *neurocardiogenic syncope* does not feature a fast pulse rate.

> ## *Neurocardiogenic Syncope*
> - *Mainly young adult women or children*
> - *Normal pulse rate during standing*
> - *Can be associated with several non-specific associated problems (inability to tolerate prolonged standing, heat intolerance, fatigue, chest pain, heart "flip-flops," exercise intolerance)*
> - *Variable outlook, can improve*
> - *Not life-threatening*

Tilt-table testing can provoke a sudden fall in blood pressure, called *neurally mediated hypotension,* in patients with *POTS* or *neurocardiogenic syncope.* Regardless of the diagnosis, acute *neurally mediated syncope* may have the same mechanism. According to one proposal, the mechanism is from marked decreases in *sympathetic nervous system* outflow to the skeletal muscle in the limbs and probably several body organs, combined with increases in *adrenomedullary hormonal system* outflow and therefore high plasma *adrenaline (epinephrine)* levels.

The combination of loss of *sympathetic vasoconstrictor tone* and *epinephrine (adrenaline)*-induced relaxation of blood vessels in skeletal muscle could decrease *vascular resistance* in skeletal muscle and in the body as a whole. It has been suggested that this combination explains the decreased *total peripheral resistance,* without a compensatory increase in the ejection of blood by the heart, the *cardiac output.* This combination characterizes *neurocardiogenic syncope.* Because of the fall in *total peripheral resistance,* without an increase in *cardiac output,* the *blood pressure* falls. The patient feels faint *(presyncope)* or actually loses consciousness *(syncope).*

Although physiological and hormonal changes that accompany *neurocardiogenic syncope* have received considerable research attention, studies so far have failed to identify predisposing factors. A decrease in the rate of *sympathetic nerve traffic* to the heart, or a restraint on release of *norepinephrine* from *sympathetic nerve terminals* in the heart, might cause a tendency to faint, by preventing compensatory increases in the force and rate of the heartbeat in response to a fall in *total peripheral resistance;* however, no published study so far has tested this idea.

Reports about a high frequency of *neurocardiogenic syncope* and *neurally mediated hypotension* during provocative *tilt table testing* have supported the view that *chronic fatigue syndrome* often includes and may result from a form of *dysautonomia.*

The usual treatments for *neurocardiogenic syncope* are the same as for *POTS:* Florinef™ and liberal salt and water intake; *β-adrenoceptor blockers; midodrine;* calf muscle resistance training; exercise training; or insertion of a pacemaker.

Consistent with the notion that decreased *sympathetic nerve traffic* or decreased *norepinephrine* release predisposes to *neurocardiogenic syncope,* some patients note improvement with sympathomimetic amines such as *d-amphetamine* or *methylphenidate (Ritalin™).*

As in *POTS,* in *neurocardiogenic syncope,* there does not seem to be much risk of chronic cardiovascular disease.

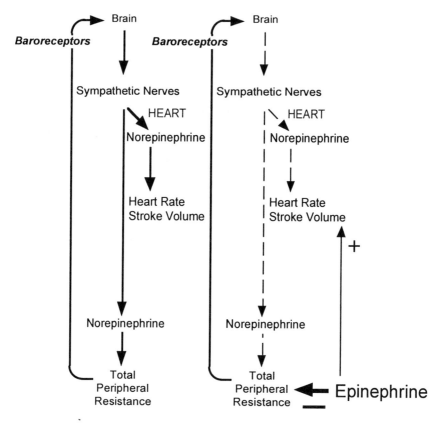

NORMAL   NEUROCARDIOGENIC
SYNCOPE

*Neurocardiogenic syncope involves an
unusual pattern where before the acute
episode, epinephrine (adrenaline) levels are
high, and yet the sympathetic nervous
system shuts down.*

Tests for Dysautonomias

There are four types of tests doctors use to diagnose dysautonomias—physiological, neuropharmacologic, neurochemical, and neuroimaging.

Physiological tests involve measurements of a body function in response to a manipulation such as standing, tilt-table-testing, or a change in room temperature.

Neuropharmacologic tests involve giving a drug and measuring its immediate effects.

Neurochemical tests involve measuring levels of body chemicals, such as the *catecholamines, norepinephrine* and *epinephrine,* either under resting conditions or in response to *physiological* or *neuropharmacologic* manipulations.

Neuroimaging tests involve actually visualizing parts of the *autonomic nervous system,* such as the *sympathetic* nerves in the heart.

This section describes examples of each type of test. Each type has its own advantages and disadvantages. Most centers that carry out *autonomic function testing* use more than one type of test, but none use all of the tests described in this section.

Physiological tests usually are simple, quick, painless, and safe. The main problem with them is that there are always several steps between the brain's directing a change in nerve traffic in the *autonomic nervous system* and the *physiological* changes that are supposed to measure the *autonomic* changes. As a result, the results of *physiological* tests are always complex and **indirect**, and they may or may not identify a problem correctly.

Neuropharmacologic tests are relatively simple and quick, but they depend on drug effects on how the patient feels or how the body functions. This means that there always is at least some risk of **side effects**. In addition, neuropharmacologic tests are somewhat complex and indirect. For instance, a neuropharmacologic test of the role of the *sympathetic nervous system* in a person's high blood pressure might include measuring the effects of a drug that blocks *sympathetic nerve traffic* on blood pressure, because a large fall in blood pressure would suggest an important role of the *sympathetic nervous system* in keeping the blood pressure high. But if blocking the *sympathetic nerve traffic* activated another system compensatorily that also increases blood pressure, then the sympathetic blocking drug might not decrease the pressure, and the doctor might mistakenly think that the *sympathetic nervous system* wasn't involved with the patient's high blood pressure.

Neurochemical tests involve measurements of levels of compounds such as *norepinephrine* in body fluids such as *plasma.* These tests can be done while the patient is at rest lying down, during a *physiological* manipulation such as exercise or tilting on a *tilt-table,* or during a *neuropharmacologic* manipulation such as blockade of *sympathetic nerve traffic* by a drug. *Neurochemical* tests themselves are safe, but the type of body fluid sampling, such as *arterial blood sampling* or *cerebrospinal fluid* sampling after a *lumbar puncture,* can involve some risk.

A major disadvantage of *neurochemical* testing is that there is **no test of parasympathetic nervous system activity.** This is because *acetylcholine,* the chemical messenger of the *parasympathetic nervous system,* is broken down by enzymes almost as soon as it enters body fluids such as the *plasma.*

Neurochemical testing based on *plasma norepinephrine* levels also can be problematic, because those levels are determined not only by the rate of entry of *norepinephrine* into the plasma but also the rate of removal *(clearance)* of *norepinephrine* from the *plasma.* In addition, *plasma norepinephrine levels* are determined complexly by a variety of processes in the *sympathetic nerve terminals. Neurochemical* testing by *plasma norepinephrine* levels requires a carefully **controlled testing situation** and **expert technical analysis** and **interpretation.** Few clinical laboratories measure *plasma* levels of *catecholamines* such as *norepinephrine* and *epinephrine,* and **laboratories vary** in the validity of the assay methods they use.

Neuroimaging tests, which are relatively new, involve actually depicting the *autonomic nerve supply* in body organs such as the heart. As yet there is no accepted neuroimaging test to visualize *parasympathetic nerve terminals.* *Sympathetic neuroimaging* is done in relatively **few centers,** and although this type of testing can produce striking images of the *sympathetic innervation* of the heart, this provides **anatomic** information about whether *sympathetic nerve terminals* are present, and it is still unclear whether *sympathetic neuroimaging* can provide information about whether those terminals are functioning normally or not.

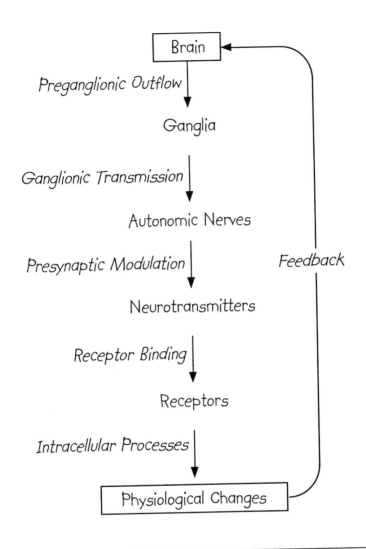

Brain

Preganglionic Outflow

Ganglia

Ganglionic Transmission

Autonomic Nerves

Presynaptic Modulation

Neurotransmitters

Receptor Binding

Receptors

Intracellular Processes

Physiological Changes

Feedback

Physiological tests involve measurement of a body function, such as pulse rate or blood pressure.

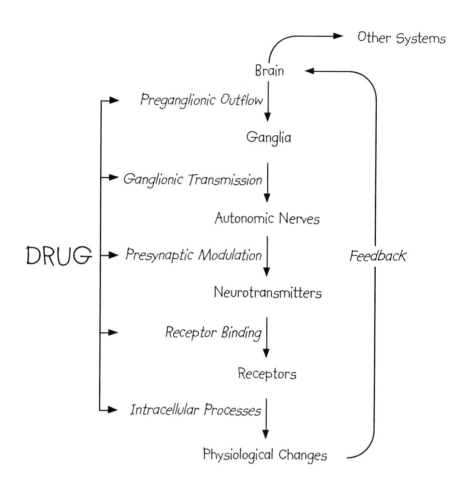

Other Systems

Brain

Preganglionic Outflow

Ganglia

Ganglionic Transmission

Autonomic Nerves

DRUG

Presynaptic Modulation

Neurotransmitters

Feedback

Receptor Binding

Receptors

Intracellular Processes

Physiological Changes

Neuropharmacologic tests involve using a drug that affects a function of the nervous system.

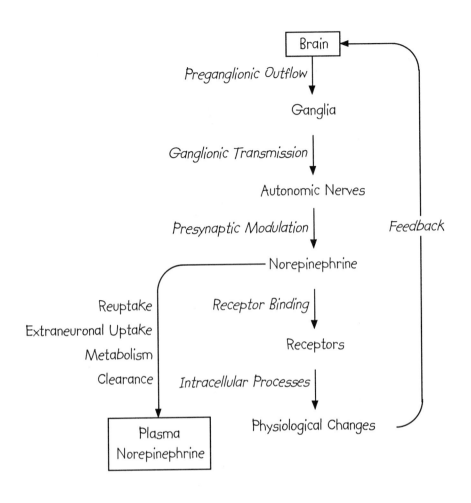

Neurochemical tests involve measuring a chemical produced in the nervous system, such as norepinephrine, the chemical messenger of the sympathetic nervous system.

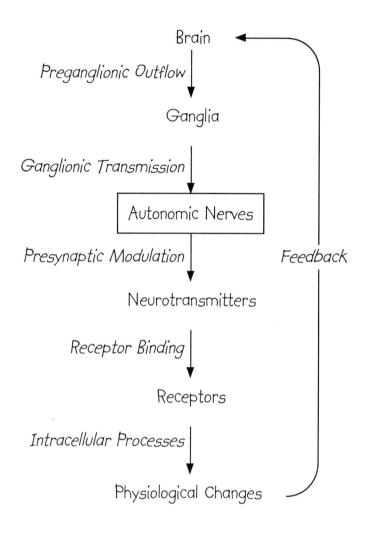

Brain

Preganglionic Outflow

Ganglia

Ganglionic Transmission

Autonomic Nerves

Presynaptic Modulation

Neurotransmitters

Receptor Binding

Receptors

Intracellular Processes

Physiological Changes

Feedback

Neuroimaging tests involve visualizing part of the nervous system, such as the autonomic nervous system.

Physiological Tests
The Valsalva Maneuver

Despite its apparent simplicity, the *Valsalva* maneuver test is one of the most important clinical physiological tests for *autonomic failure*.

In the Valsalva maneuver, the patient blows against a resistance for several seconds and then relaxes.

The maneuver consists of blowing against a resistance for several seconds and then relaxing. Often the patient blows into a tube connected to a blood pressure gauge, moving the gauge's needle to a particular pressure and keeping the needle there for 10-15 seconds.

The instant the patient begins to blow, the sudden increase in chest and abdominal pressure forces blood out of the chest and down the arms. This increases blood pressure briefly (Phase I of the maneuver). The increase in blood pressure in Phase I is mechanical and not part of a reflex.

Soon afterwards, however, the amount of blood ejected by the heart with each beat *(stroke volume)* plummets, because the straining decreases entry of blood from the veins into the heart. Blood pressure progressively falls (Phase II). The brain immediately senses this fall, due to decreased input to the brain from stretch receptors *(baroreceptors)* in the walls of the heart and major blood vessels. The brain directs a rapid increase in outflows in the *sympathetic nervous system* to the blood vessels and a rapid decrease in outflow in the *parasympathetic nervous system* to the heart. The increase in *sympathetic nerve traffic* leads to more release of *norepinephrine* from the nerve terminals, and the released *norepinephrine* tightens blood vessels throughout the body. The *total peripheral resistance* to blood flow in the body goes up, just like tightening the nozzle at the end of a garden hose increases the pressure in the hose. Therefore, normally, at the end of Phase II the blood pressure increases from its minimum value, even though the amount of blood ejected by the heart remains low.

When the patient relaxes at the end of the maneuver, briefly the blood pressure falls (Phase III)—a mirror image of the brief increase in Phase I. Blood rushes back into the chest, and within a few heartbeats the heart ejects this blood. The blood pressure increases (Phase IV). Since the blood vessels are constricted, the normal amount of filling of the constricted vessels produces an overshoot of blood pressure, just as pressure in a garden hose attains higher levels if one turns on the faucet with the nozzle tightened. Finally, in response to this Phase IV overshoot of blood pressure, *sympathetic nervous system* outflow to blood vessels falls and *parasympathetic* outflow to the heart increases. This causes a rapid return of blood pressure and heart rate to normal.

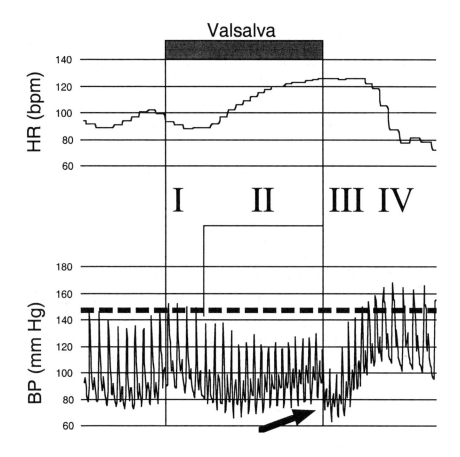

Normal blood pressure (BP) and heart rate (HR) responses to the Valsalva maneuver.

In a patient with sympathetic neurocirculatory failure, during Phase II the blood vessels fail to constrict reflexively, and so blood pressure falls progressively and does not increase toward baseline at the end of Phase II.

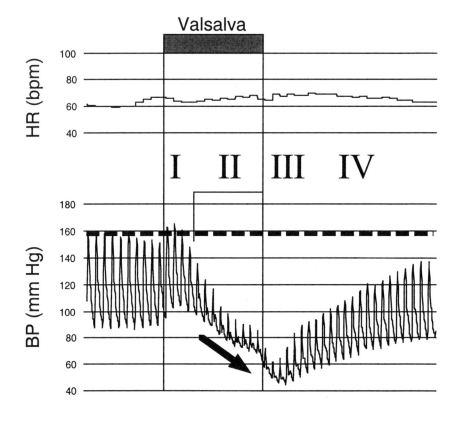

Abnormal blood pressure (BP) and heart rate (HR) responses to the Valsalva maneuver, indicating parasympathetic and sympathetic nervous system failure.

During Phase IV, because of the lack of tightening of blood vessels, there is no rapid increase in blood pressure and no Phase IV overshoot of pressure. Instead, the blood pressure gradually increases slowly back to the baseline value.

The responses of pulse rate to the *Valsalva maneuver* depend mainly on changes in *parasympathetic nervous system* outflow to the heart via the *vagus* nerve. In Phase II, the pulse rate increases, and in Phase IV the pulse rate returns rapidly to baseline. In *parasympathetic neurocirculatory failure* or *baroreflex failure,* the pulse rate remains unchanged both during and after performance of the maneuver.

Note that one must monitor the beat-to-beat blood pressure changes in order to diagnose *sympathetic neurocirculatory failure* based on the *Valsalva* maneuver. Until recently, such monitoring required insertion of a catheter into an artery. Since neurologists rarely feel comfortable doing this, they usually settle for recording only the peak and trough pulse rates during and after performance of the maneuver. This may enable a diagnosis of *parasympathetic neurocirculatory failure* but cannot diagnose *sympathetic neurocirculatory failure.*

The recent introduction of special testing devices has provided non-invasive means to follow blood pressure beat-to-beat and detection of *sympathetic neurocirculatory failure.*

Forearm Blood Flow

This non-invasive test measures the rate of blood flow in the forearm. From the *forearm blood flow (FBF)* and the blood pressure *(mean arterial pressure, MAP)*, the *forearm vascular resistance (FVR)* can be estimated. In the garden hose analogy, the *FVR* would correspond to the extent of tightening of the nozzle. One of the main ways the body has to regulate blood pressure is by regulating *vascular resistance,* using the *sympathetic nervous system.*

When a person stands up or is tilted on a tilt table as part of *tilt-table testing,* the amount of blood ejected by the heart per minute falls, due to the force of gravity, which tends to pool blood in the legs and lower abdomen and decreases *venous return* to the heart. The brain directs an increase in sympathetic nervous system outflows, which increases *peripheral resistance* to blood flow and helps keep the average *blood pressure (mean arterial pressure)* normal, despite the decrease in *cardiac output.*

To measure *forearm blood flow,* a blood pressure cuff is attached around the upper arm, and a special bracelet-like device called a *strain gauge* is attached around the upper forearm. The *strain gauge* measures stretch very sensitively. For a measurement of forearm blood flow, the blood pressure cuff is inflated to just above the *venous pressure* but below the *arterial pressure.*

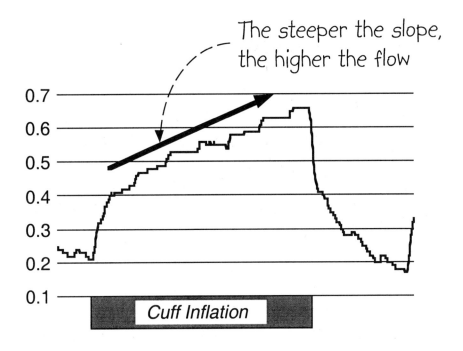

The steeper the slope, the higher the flow

Cuff Inflation

Resistance = Pressure / Flow
FVR = MAP / FBF
TPR = MAP / CO

Blood flow in a limb can be measured non-invasively using a blood pressure cuff and a bracelet-like device around the limb.

This is like tightening a tourniquet around the upper arm, for obtaining a blood sample. Because the cuff pressure is above the *venous pressure,* blood in the forearm and hand can't get past the cuff, and because the cuff pressure is below the *arterial pressure,* blood can still enter the forearm and hand. In this situation, the volume of the forearm expands slightly, and the *strain gauge* senses the increase in volume. If the rate of blood flow into the forearm is high, then the volume of the forearm increases rapidly after the cuff is inflated; and if the rate of blood flow is low, then the volume of the forearm increases more slowly. By a simple calculation we can estimate the blood flow into the forearm, from the rate of increase in the volume of the forearm after the cuff is inflated. Usually, measurement of *forearm blood flow* is done at least five times, to obtain a reliable average value.

Once the rate of *forearm blood flow (FBF)* is known, the *forearm vascular resistance (FVR)* can be estimated from the average blood pressure *(mean arterial pressure, MAP)* divided by the *forearm blood flow.* This is a similar calculation as for measuring *total peripheral resistance (TPR)* from the *mean arterial pressure (MAP)* divided by the *cardiac output (CO).* When a person stands up or is tilted on a tilt-table as part of *tilt-table testing,* the *forearm vascular resistance* normally increases. A failure of the *forearm vascular resistance* to increase during standing is a sign of *sympathetic neurocirculatory failure.*

Incidentally, the logo of the National Dysautonomia Research Foundation is based on the signal used to measure *forearm vascular resistance.* Just before a patient faints, the *forearm blood flow* increases. The logo shows the increase in the *forearm blood flow* on repeated measurements, as in the background the patient's skin color turns from a healthy red color to a deathly blue!

Power Spectral Analysis of Heart Rate Variability

This test is much simpler than the fancy name suggests. Normally, a person's heart rate is not constant. The pulse rate increases when the person breathes in and then decreases when the person breathes out. This means that the pulse rate normally oscillates in a wave-like pattern.

The change in pulse rate from breathing is sometimes called *respiratory sinus arrhythmia.* This sounds like an abnormal heart rhythm, but it actually is a sign of a healthy heart. *Respiratory sinus arrhythmia* is thought to result from changes in *parasympathetic nervous system* influences on the heart.

If one graphs the size of the oscillation as a function of the frequency of the heartbeats, then at the frequency of breathing, there is a peak of *"power."* In people who have failure of the *parasympathetic nervous system*, there is little or no *respiratory sinus arrhythmia,* and there is no peak of *power* at the frequency of breathing. This sort of analysis has revealed a second peak of *power,* at a lower frequency than the frequency of breathing.

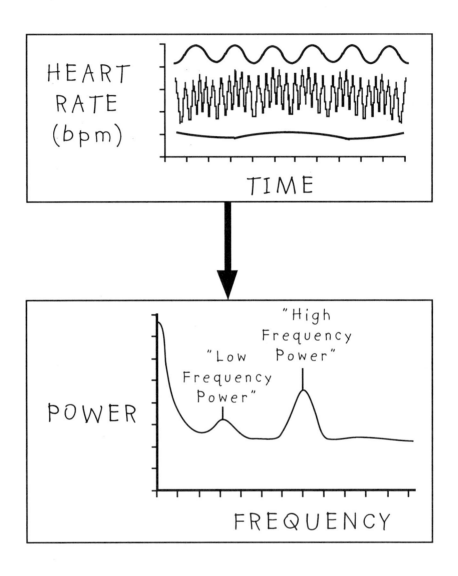

Power spectral analysis is a non-invasive way to interpret heart rate changes.

Researchers have thought that this low frequency *power* is related to *sympathetic nervous system* influences on the heart.

Power spectral analysis of heart rate offers the advantages of being safe, technically easy, and fast. The main disadvantage is that the meaning of *low frequency power* as an index of *sympathetic nervous system* activity in the heart remains in dispute.

Tilt-Table Testing

Tilt-table testing is done to see if standing up *(orthostasis)* provokes a sudden fall in blood pressure *(neurally mediated hypotension),* an excessive increase in pulse rate *(postural tachycardia syndrome, POTS),* or fainting *(neurally mediated syncope).*

> *Tilt-table testing is used to detect POTS or neurocardiogenic syncope.*

The testing itself is simple. The patient lies on a stretcher-like table, straps like seat belts are attached around the abdomen and legs, and the patient is tilted upright at an angle. The exact angle used varies from center to center and may be from 60 degrees to 90 degrees. The tilting goes on for up to many minutes (this again varies from center to center) up to about 45 minutes. If the patient tolerates the tilting for this period, then the patient may receive a drug, such as *isoproterenol* or *nitroglycerine,* which might provoke a sudden fall in blood pressure or loss of consciousness. As soon as the test becomes positive, the patient is put back into a position lying flat or with the head down, and sometimes fluid is given by vein. Patients usually recover consciousness within a minute or two.

Tilt-table testing is a form of *provocative* test. The doctors are hoping to reproduce the patient's problem in a controlled laboratory situation. The testing is quite safe when done by experienced personnel, in a setting where emergency backup is available.

There are several disadvantages of *tilt-table testing.* One is the issue of *false-positive* results, especially when a drug such as *isoproterenol* is used. In a *false-positive* test, the results of the test are positive, but some healthy people can have a positive test result, so that a positive test result might not actually mean that anything really is "wrong."

Another disadvantage is that most *tilt-table testing* does not provide information about disease mechanisms. This means that, beyond verifying the patient's complaints, the testing does little or nothing to suggest treatments that might be effective.

Tilt-table testing is not useful in patients with a persistent fall in blood pressure each time they stand up *(orthostatic hypotension),* because the results are a foregone conclusion: the blood pressure will fall progressively beginning as soon as the tilting starts.

Sweat Tests

Sweating is an important way people regulate body temperature in response to external heat. The brain increases sweating by directing an increase in *sympathetic nervous system* traffic to sweat glands in the skin. The chemical messenger, *acetylcholine,* is released, and the *acetylcholine* acts on the sweat glands to stimulate production of sweat.

> *Sweat tests evaluate a particular part of "automatic" nervous system function.*

There are several ways to measure *sympathetic cholinergic* sweating in response to external heat *(thermoregulatory sweat test, TST)*. One is from sprinkling starch with iodine all over the body. When the starch-iodine combination is wetted, the powder turns brown. One can then photograph the body and see which parts sweated. Sometimes other powder-dye combinations are used. When the skin becomes sweaty, the ability to conduct electricity increases dramatically, because of the salt and water in the sweat, and one can monitor the electrical conductivity. Sweat increases local humidity, and one can also monitor the humidity in a chamber attached to the skin.

Another way to test sweating is from the *galvanic skin response (GSR)* or *skin sympathetic test (SST)*. The *galvanic skin response* is part of polygraphic "lie detector" testing. When a person is suddenly distressed, or a small electric shock is delivered, increased activities of the *sympathetic nervous system* and the *adrenomedullary hormonal system* evoke sweating. One can also measure sweating from humidity in a capsule applied to the skin.

Advantages of sweat tests are that they are generally safe, simple, and quick. A disadvantage is that they only measure *physiological* changes as a result of release of *acetylcholine* from *sympathetic nerve terminals* or *epinephrine* from the *adrenal gland.* There are *dysautonomias* where the patient has normal sweating.

Another disadvantage is that sweat tests are only indirectly and complexly related to activity of the *sympathetic nervous system,* and they provide little information about the exact mechanism of the *dysautonomia.*

The Cold Pressor Test

In the *cold pressor test,* the patient dunks a hand into ice-cold water. This rapidly increases the blood pressure, by increasing activity of the *sympathetic nervous system.* Since the test involves not only cold but also pain, the *cold pressor test* can only be done for a minute or two. A similar limitation applies for isometric handgrip exercise.

Neuropharmacologic Tests

QSART

"QSART" stands for *"Quantitative Sudomotor Axon Reflex Test."*

> *The QSART is a special form of sweat test.*

This test is a form of sweat test. Sweating in response to altered environmental temperature results from the effects of the chemical messenger, *acetylcholine,* released from *sympathetic nerve terminals* near sweat glands in the skin. This arrangement is different from that for alterations in the pulse rate and blood pressure that result from effects of *norepinephrine* released from *sympathetic nerve terminals* in the heart and blood vessel walls. The *QSART* is a test of the ability of *sympathetic nerve terminals* in the skin to release *acetylcholine* and increase sweat production.

As in some other sweat tests, in the *QSART* procedure, dried nitrogen (or dried air, or air with a known amount of humidity) is pumped at a controlled rate through a small plastic, dome-like capsule placed on the skin. When the person sweats, the humidity in the chamber increases, as the sweat droplets evaporate. This provides a rapid measure of sweat production. For *QSART* testing,

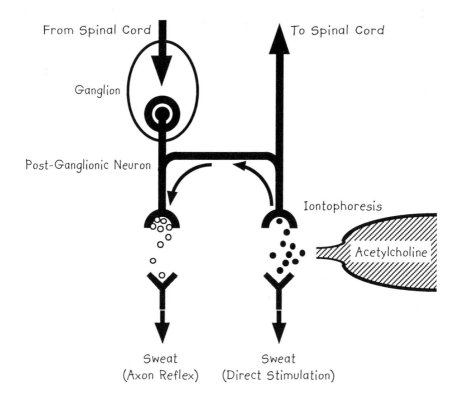

From Spinal Cord

To Spinal Cord

Ganglion

Post-Ganglionic Neuron

Iontophoresis

Acetylcholine

Sweat
(Axon Reflex)

Sweat
(Direct Stimulation)

Diagram of the QSART test.

a drug that stimulates *acetylcholine receptors* (for instance *acetylcholine* itself) is applied to a nearby patch of skin, by a special procedure called *iontophoresis.* The locally applied *acetylcholine* evokes sweating at the site where it is given, but in addition, by way of a type of reflex called an *axon reflex, sympathetic nerve terminals* under the nearby plastic capsule release the body's own *acetylcholine,* resulting in sweat production measured by increased humidity in the capsule.

If a person had a loss of *sympathetic nerve terminals* that release *acetylcholine* (loss of *cholinergic* terminals), then applying *acetylcholine* to the patch of skin near the test capsule would not lead to increased sweating or increased humidity in the test capsule. On the other hand, if the person had intact *sympathetic cholinergic nerve terminals,* then applying acetylcholine to a patch of skin near the test capsule would increase the humidity in the capsule. If the person had a brain disease that prevented increases in *sympathetic nerve traffic* during exposure to increased environmental temperature, then the person would not be able to increase the humidity in the capsule in response to an increase in the room temperature, and yet the person would have a normal *QSART* response.

By this sort of *neuropharmacologic* test, doctors can distinguish *sympathetic cholinergic failure* due to loss of *cholinergic terminals* from failure due to abnormal regulation of *sympathetic nerve traffic* to intact *cholinergic terminals.*

Advantages of the *QSART* are that it is generally safe, quick, quantitative, and easy for a technician to perform. There are also several disadvantages. The equipment required is fairly expensive, and relatively few centers have *QSART* testing available, so that **availability** of the test is an issue. As in other tests where the key factor being measured is *physiological* (in this case, sweat production), the results are **indirect**. For instance, a problem with the ability to make *acetylcholine* in the nerve terminals or with the ability of acetylcholine to bind to its *receptors* in the sweat glands would result in the same abnormal *QSART* responses as if the *sympathetic cholinergic terminals* were lost. Finally, *QSART* results may or may not identify problems in regulation of the heart and blood vessels by other parts of the *autonomic nervous system.* In other words, the *QSART* results might not be **representative**.

Trimethaphan Infusion Test

Trimethaphan is a type of drug called a *ganglion blocker.*

In the *autonomic nervous system,* control signals from the brain and spinal cord are relayed through the *ganglia,* and nerves from the *ganglia, postganglionic* nerves, deliver those signals to the *nerve terminals* near or in the target tissues. The control signals are relayed in the *ganglia* by release of the chemical messenger, *acetylcholine,* which binds to specific receptors on the *postganglionic* cells, called *nicotinic receptors.*

Stimulation of the *nicotinic receptors,* such as by *nicotine* itself, *increases postganglionic nerve traffic* in both the *parasympathetic nervous system* and the *sympathetic nervous system.*

Trimethaphan does just the opposite. It blocks *nicotinic receptors* in the *ganglia.* By blocking the *receptors, trimethaphan* blocks the transmission of nerve impulses in the *ganglia* to the *postganglionic nerves* of the *sympathetic nervous system* and *parasympathetic nervous system.* The rates of *sympathetic nerve traffic* and *parasympathetic nerve traffic* fall to virtually zero.

Because of the blockade of transmission of nerve impulses in *ganglia, trimethaphan* normally produces clear effects on a variety of body functions. When a person stands up, the ability to maintain blood pressure depends importantly on reflexes that tighten blood vessels, by way of increased *sympathetic nerve traffic. Trimethaphan* therefore always produces a fall in blood pressure when the person stands up, called *orthostatic hypotension.* If the person is lying down at the time, then *trimethaphan* produces a relatively small decrease in blood pressure. Probably the most noticeable effect of *trimethaphan* in someone who is lying down is a dry mouth. This is because of blockade of the *parasympathetic nervous system,* which is responsible for production of watery saliva.

In the *trimethaphan infusion test,* the drug is given by vein at a dose calculated so as not to decrease the blood pressure excessively. The blood pressure and pulse rate are monitored frequently or continuously, and blood may be sampled from an indwelling catheter in an arm vein, for measurements of *plasma norepinephrine levels* or levels of other neurochemicals.

If a patient had *autonomic failure* due to a loss of *sympathetic nerve terminals,* such as in *Parkinson's disease with orthostatic hypotension,* there would be no release of *norepinephrine* from the nerve terminals, because of the absence of the terminals. *Trimethaphan* in such a patient would not affect the blood pressure. But if a patient had *autonomic failure* due to a brain disease, such as the *Shy-Drager syndrome (multiple system atrophy with sympathetic neurocirculatory failure),* where there was an inability to regulate *sympathetic nerve traffic* to intact terminals, there might be ongoing, unregulated release of *norepinephrine* from the nerve terminals. *Trimethaphan* in such a patient would decrease the blood pressure.

The *trimethaphan infusion test* therefore can provide information about whether *autonomic failure* is associated with a loss of *sympathetic nerve terminals* or from failure of the brain to regulate *sympathetic nerve traffic* appropriately.

In some patients with long-term high blood pressure *(hypertension),* the *hypertension* seems to reflect an overall increase in the rate of nerve traffic in the *sympathetic nervous system.* This increases delivery of *norepinephrine* to its *receptors* in the heart and blood vessels, causing an increase in the output of blood by the

Parkinson's Disease with Orthostatic Hypotension

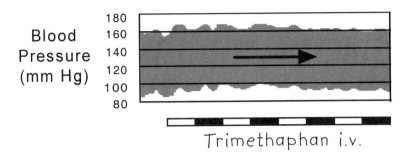

Blood Pressure (mm Hg)

Trimethaphan i.v.

Shy-Drager Syndrome

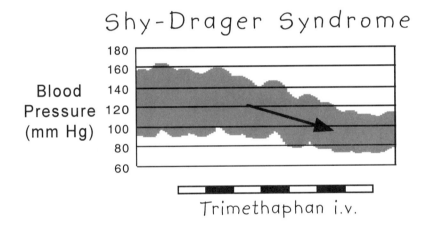

Blood Pressure (mm Hg)

Trimethaphan i.v.

The trimethaphan infusion test can help to identify different causes of autonomic failure.

heart *(cardiac output)* and tightening of blood vessels *(vasoconstriction)*. By either or both mechanisms, the blood pressure would be high because of the high rate of delivery of *norepinephrine* to its receptors. Some investigators have called this *hypernoradrenergic hypertension.* In a patient with *hypernoradrenergic hypertension,* infusion of *trimethaphan* would be expected to decrease the rate of *norepinephrine* release from the *sympathetic nerve terminals,* and the extent of the fall in the *plasma norepinephrine level* would be related to the extent of the fall in blood pressure. In a patient with an equal amount of hypertension, but with a normal rate of nerve traffic in the *sympathetic nervous system, trimethaphan* would not be expected to decrease the blood pressure as much.

Because *trimethaphan* is a potent blocker of the *sympathetic nervous system* and the *parasympathetic nervous system,* the drug must be given at a carefully controlled rate, by personnel who are well acquainted with its effects. If the dose is too high, then the blood pressure (especially the *systolic* blood pressure) can fall too much. The effects of *trimethaphan* wear off quickly after the infusion is stopped, and so if too much drug is being given, decreasing the infusion rate or stopping the infusion will eliminate the side effects within minutes. An antidote drug should be available that directly stimulates *norepinephrine receptors.* Sometimes *trimethaphan* can evoke release of *histamine,* which can produce itching, wheezing, or decreased blood blood pressure. An anti-histamine drug should also be available.

Yohimbine Challenge Test

Yohimbine is a type of drug called an *alpha-2 adrenoceptor blocker. Alpha-2 adrenoceptors* are *receptors* for *norepinephrine* that exist at high concentrations in certain parts of the brain, on *sympathetic nerve terminals,* and in blood vessel walls.

When *alpha-2 adrenoceptors* in the brain are blocked, this increases *sympathetic nerve traffic. Alpha-2 adrenoceptors* on *sympathetic nerve terminals* act like a brake on *norepinephrine* release from the terminals. When *alpha-2 adrenoceptors* on *sympathetic nerve terminals* are blocked, this increases the amount of *norepinephrine* release for a given amount of *sympathetic nerve traffic.* Yohimbine, by blocking *alpha-2 adrenoceptors* in the brain and on *sympathetic nerve terminals,* therefore releases *norepinephrine* from the terminals. The released norepinephrine binds to *alpha-1 adrenoceptors* in blood vessel walls, causing an increase in blood pressure.

Because of the blockade of *alpha-2 adrenoceptors* in the brain, *yohimbine* can produce any of several **behavioral or emotional effects,** which vary from person to person. *Yohimbine* can cause an increase in alertness or feelings such as anxiety or sadness, or, on the other hand, happiness or a sense of energy. Rarely, yohimbine can cause a panic attack.

Yohimbine usually causes *trembling,* which sometimes is so severe that the teeth chatter, and it sometimes also causes **paleness** of the skin, **goosebumps**, and **hair standing out,** as if the person were either very cold or distressed. Actually, the body temperature does not fall at all, and the person does not feel cold. Another sometimes noticeable effect of *yohimbine* is an **increase in salivation.** This is probably because of an increase in the rate of *sympathetic nerve traffic* to the *salivary glands.*

In the *yohimbine challenge test,* the drug is given by vein for several minutes or given by mouth as a single dose. *Yohimbine* given by vein is currently an investigational drug. The blood pressure and pulse rate are monitored frequently or continuously, and blood often is sampled from an indwelling catheter in an arm vein, for measurements of *plasma norepinephrine levels* or levels of other neurochemicals.

If a patient had *autonomic failure* due to a loss of *sympathetic nerve terminals,* such as in *Parkinson's disease with orthostatic hypotension,* there would be no release of *norepinephrine* from the nerve terminals, regardless of the nerve traffic, because of the absence of the terminals. *Yohimbine* in such a patient would not affect the blood pressure. But if a patient had *autonomic failure* due to a brain disease, such as the *Shy-Drager syndrome (multiple system atrophy with sympathetic neurocirculatory failure),* where there was an inability to regulate *sympathetic nerve traffic* to intact terminals, *yohimbine* would increase the blood pressure, and

Parkinson's Disease with Orthostatic Hypotension

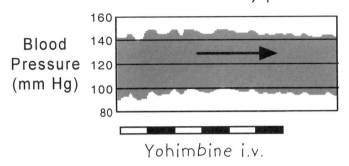

Blood Pressure (mm Hg)

Yohimbine i.v.

Shy-Drager Syndrome

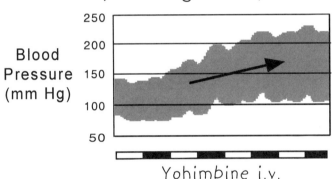

Blood Pressure (mm Hg)

Yohimbine i.v.

The yohimbine challenge test can help to identify different causes of autonomic failure.

because of the inability to regulate *sympathetic nerve traffic,* the brain would not reflexively decrease the *sympathetic nerve traffic* to compensate for the increased blood pressure. This means that infusion of yohimbine into such a patient might produce a large increase in blood pressure. If the patient already had high blood pressure, or if the doctor already strongly suspected a disease such as the *Shy-Drager syndrome,* then the dose would be decreased, or the doctor might decide that carrying out the test would not be worth the risk.

In some patients with long-term high blood pressure *(hypertension),* the *hypertension* seems to reflect an overall increase in the rate of nerve traffic in the *sympathetic nervous system.* This increases delivery of *norepinephrine* to its *receptors* in the heart and blood vessels, causing an increase in the output of blood by the heart *(cardiac output)* and tightening of blood vessels *(vasoconstriction).* By either or both mechanisms, the blood pressure is high because of the high rate of delivery of *norepinephrine* to its receptors. Some investigators have called this *hypernoradrenergic hypertension.*

In patients with *hypernoradrenergic hypertension,* some of the released *norepinephrine* binds to the *alpha-2 adrenoceptors* on the *sympathetic nerve terminals,* and this puts a brake on the *norepinephrine* release. Infusion of *yohimbine* by vein into such patients increases both blood pressure and the *plasma norepinephrine level,* by blocking this restraint. The finding of a large increase in blood pressure coupled with a large increase in the *plasma norepinephrine level* provides support for the diagnosis of *hypernoradrenergic hypertension.*

In patients who have decreased activity of the *cell membrane norepinephrine transporter,* or *NET,* when *yohimbine* releases *norepinephrine* from the *sympathetic nerve terminals,* the released *norepinephrine* is not inactivated by "recycling" of the *norepinephrine* back into the nerve terminals. This results in excessive delivery of *norepinephrine* to its *receptors,* both in the brain and outside the brain. In patients with NET deficiency, *yohimbine* therefore produces a large increase in the *plasma norepinephrine level* and large increases in the pulse rate and blood pressure. *Yohimbine* can also evoke *panic* or chest pain or pressure that can mimic the chest pain or pressure in *coronary artery disease.*

The *yohimbine challenge test* therefore can provide information about whether *autonomic failure* is associated with a loss of *sympathetic nerve terminals* or from failure of the brain to regulate *sympathetic nerve traffic* appropriately. The test can also be used to identify *hypernoradrenergic hypertension* or *NET deficiency.* The effects of *yohimbine* wear off over several minutes, once the infusion ends. If the blood pressure increase were excessive, the quickest way to bring the pressure down would be to stop the infusion and, if the patient had *orthostatic hypotension,* have the patient stand up. Very rarely, an antidote drug that stimulates *alpha-2 adrenoceptors,* such as *clonidine,* has to be given.

Because *yohimbine* given by vein is an investigational drug that produces important effects on functions of the *sympathetic nervous system,* the *yohimbine challenge test* should be done only by personnel who are well acquainted with its effects.

Clonidine Suppression Test

Clonidine stimulates *alpha-2 adrenoceptors* in the brain, on *sympathetic nerve terminals,* and in blood vessel walls. When *alpha-2 adrenoceptors* in the brain are stimulated, this decreases *sympathetic nerve traffic, and* when *alpha-2 adrenoceptors* on *sympathetic nerve terminals* are stimulated, this decreases the amount of *norepinephrine* release for a given amount of *sympathetic nerve traffic.*

Released *norepinephrine* binds to both *alpha-2 adrenoceptors* and *alpha-1 adrenoceptors* in blood vessel walls. Even though *clonidine* stimulates *alpha-2 adrenoceptors,* which would constrict blood vessels, the drug is so powerful in decreasing release of *norepinephrine* that normally after a dose of *clonidine* the blood pressure falls. *Clonidine* is an approved drug for the treatment of long-term high blood pressure *(hypertension).*

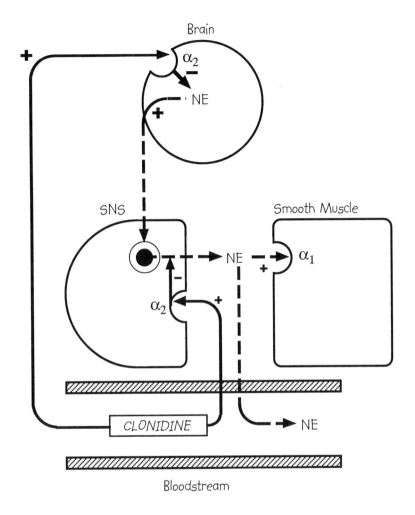

The clonidine suppression test can be helpful in identifying causes of abnormal levels of norepinephrine (NE), the chemical messenger of the sympathetic nervous system (SNS).

By stimulating *alpha-2 adrenoceptors* in the brain, *clonidine* usually produces some sedation. It can cause a decrease in alertness or a decrease in the sense of energy. *Clonidine* is effective in relieving symptoms of withdrawal from alcohol or opiate-type narcotics.

Clonidine can produce a dry mouth and a small decrease in the pulse rate. This is probably because of a decrease in the rate of *sympathetic nerve traffic* to the *salivary glands* and heart.

In the *clonidine suppression test,* the drug is given by mouth, usually at a dose of 300 micrograms, which would be the total amount of the drug given in divided doses in a day. The blood pressure and pulse rate are monitored over the course of a few hours, and blood is sampled from an indwelling catheter in an arm vein, for measurements of *plasma norepinephrine levels.*

If a patient had *autonomic failure* due to a loss of *sympathetic nerve terminals,* such as in *Parkinson's disease with orthostatic hypotension,* there would be no release of *norepinephrine* from the nerve terminals, regardless of the nerve traffic, because of the absence of the terminals. *Clonidine* in such a patient would not affect the blood pressure, or it might actually increase the blood pressure, due to stimulation of *alpha-2 adrenoceptors* in the blood vessel walls.
But if a patient had *autonomic failure* due to a brain disease, such as the *Shy-Drager syndrome (multiple system atrophy with sympathetic neurocirculatory failure),* where there was an inability to regulate

sympathetic nerve traffic to intact terminals, there would be *norepinephrine* in the terminals, and *clonidine* would inhibit its release. *Clonidine* in such a patient would decrease the blood pressure, and because of the inability to regulate *sympathetic nerve traffic,* the brain would not reflexively increase the *sympathetic nerve traffic* to compensate for the decreased blood pressure. This means that *clonidine* might produce a large decrease in blood pressure.

In some patients with long-term high blood pressure *(hypertension),* the *hypertension* is associated with an overall increase in the rate of nerve traffic in the *sympathetic nervous system.* The blood pressure would be high because of the high rate of delivery of *norepinephrine* to its receptors—*hypernoradrenergic hypertension. Clonidine* binds to the *alpha-2 adrenoceptors* on the *sympathetic nerve terminals,* and this puts a brake on the *norepinephrine* release. *Clonidine* given to such patients decreases both blood pressure and the *plasma norepinephrine level.*The finding of a large decrease in blood pressure coupled with a large decrease in the *plasma norepinephrine level* provides support for the diagnosis of *hypernoradrenergic hypertension.*

Rarely, *hypernoradrenergic hypertension* results from a tumor that produces *catecholamines* such as *norepinephrine* and *epinephrine.* The tumor is called a *pheochromocytoma.* The *clonidine suppression test* is an accepted diagnostic test for *pheochromocytoma.* If the *hypernoradrenergic hypertension* resulted from a high rate of *sympathetic nerve traffic,* then *clonidine* would decrease the elevated *plasma norepinephrine level.* But if the patient had a "pheo," which would produce *catecholamines* independently of the rate of *sympathetic nerve traffic, clonidine* would fail to decrease the *plasma norepinephrine level.* In other words, in a positive *clonidine suppression test* for *pheochromocytoma,* the *plasma norepinephrine level* fails to decrease after a dose of *clonidine,* despite the presence of *hypernoradrenergic hypertension.*

The effects of *clonidine* wear off over several hours. Patients can feel sedated even up to the next day. Therefore, patients should not drive or operate heavy machinery for at least 24 hours after having a *clonidine suppression test.* The drug rarely if ever produces a dangerous fall in blood pressure.

Isoproterenol Infusion Test

Isoproterenol (brand name Isuprel™) stimulates *beta-adrenoceptors. Beta-adrenoceptor* stimulation has several important effects in the body. Stimulation of *beta-adrenoceptors* in the heart increases the rate and force of the heartbeat and therefore increases the output of blood by the heart per minute *(cardiac output).* Stimulation of *beta-adrenoceptors* in the bronchioles, the small airway tubes in the lungs, opens them and therefore can

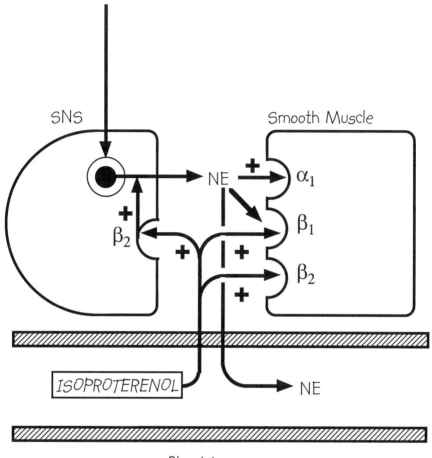

SNS

Smooth Muscle

NE

α_1

β_1

β_2

β_2

ISOPROTERENOL

NE

Bloodstream

The isoproterenol infusion test can help identify causes of abnormal heart rate or inability to tolerate prolonged standing.

reverse acute asthma attacks. Stimulation of *beta-adrenoceptors* in the liver converts stored energy in the form of *glycogen* to immediately available energy in the form of *glucose.* Stimulation of *beta-adrenoceptors* in blood vessel walls of skeletal muscle relaxes the blood vessels, decreasing the resistance to blood flow in the body as a whole *(total peripheral resistance).* Stimulation of *beta-adrenoceptors* on *sympathetic nerve terminals* increases the release of *norepinephrine.*

Isoproterenol is infused by vein as part of diagnostic testing for a few types of dysautonomias, which appear to overlap and may be different forms of the same problem. In the *hyperdynamic circulation syndrome,* the patient has a relatively fast pulse rate, high *cardiac output,* a variable blood pressure that tends to be increased, a tendency towards panic or anxiety attacks, excessive increases in pulse rate in response to *isoproterenol* given by vein, and improvement by treatment with the *beta-adrenoceptor blocker, propranolol.* The same holds true for many relatively young patients with early, borderline *hypertension.* Patients with the *postural tachycardia syndrome (POTS)* also can have a fast pulse rate, even when lying down, excessive increases in pulse rate during *isoproterenol* infusion, and sometimes panic evoked by the infusion.

Isoproterenol infusion is also done as part of tilt-table testing in patients with *chronic fatigue syndrome* or *chronic orthostatic intolerance.* After prolonged upright tilting, infusion of *isoproterenol* can bring on a rapid fall in blood pressure or loss of consciousness, converting a negative *tilt-table test* to a positive *tilt-table test*. This might arise from stimulation of the heart by *isoproterenol* or from relaxation of blood vessels in skeletal muscle, which would shunt blood away from the brain and towards the limbs.

Of course, this brings up the issue of how frequently a healthy person might have one of these reactions in response to *isoproterenol* infusion in the setting of prolonged tilting, which would be a false-positive result.

The effects of *isoproterenol* wear off rapidly within minutes of stopping the infusion. The drug does not enter the brain well, and so there are usually few if any behavioral or emotional responses. *Isoproterenol* can increase the rate or depth of respiration, produce trembling, or bring on abnormal heart rhythms or abnormal heartbeats. The risk of these side effects disappears as soon as the drug wears off. Because of the increase in pulse rate and the force of the heartbeat, *isoproterenol* infusion increases the work of the heart, and this might cause problems such as chest pressure in patients with *coronary artery disease.*

Neurochemical Tests

Neurochemical tests of *autonomic nervous system* function mainly involve the *sympathetic nervous system* or *adrenomedullary hormonal system.* This is because the main chemical messengers of these systems, *norepinephrine* and *epinephrine (adrenaline),* are relatively stable and can be measured in the plasma, while the main chemical messenger of the *parasympathetic nervous system, acetylcholine,* undergoes rapid breakdown and cannot be measured in the plasma.

Plasma Norepinephrine Levels

Since *norepinephrine* is the main chemical messenger of the *sympathetic nervous system,* doctors have often used the *plasma norepinephrine level* as an index of *sympathetic nervous system* "activity" in the body as a whole.

Plasma norepinephrine is used to test the sympathetic nervous system.

There is some validity in doing this, but the relationship between the rate of *sympathetic nerve traffic* and the concentration of *norepinephrine* in the plasma is complex and indirect and is influenced by many factors such as commonly used drugs and activities of daily life. The blood sample therefore should be obtained under carefully controlled or monitored conditions, and the *plasma norepinephrine level* should be interpreted by an expert.

Here is a brief description of some of the complexities involved:

First, only a small percent of the *norepinephrine* released from *sympathetic nerve terminals* actually makes its way into the bloodstream. Most is "recycled" back into the nerve terminals, by a process called *"Uptake-1,"* using a special transporter called the *"cell membrane norepinephrine transporter,"* or *"NET."* This means that a person might have a high *plasma norepinephrine level,* despite a normal rate of *sympathetic nerve traffic,* if the *NET* were blocked by a drug or weren't working right.

Second, the *plasma norepinephrine level* is determined not only by the rate of entry of *norepinephrine* into the plasma but also by the rate of removal of *norepinephrine* from the plasma. It happens that *norepinephrine* is cleared from the plasma extremely rapidly. This means that a person might have a high *plasma norepinephrine level* because of a problem with the ability to remove *norepinephrine* from the plasma, such as in kidney failure.

Third, *norepinephrine* is produced in *sympathetic nerve terminals* by the action of three enzymes (*tyrosine hydroxylase,* or *TH, DOPA decarboxylase,* or *DDC,* and *dopamine-beta-hydroxylase,* or *DBH*), along with other required chemicals such as vitamin C, vitamin B6, and oxygen. In addition, *norepinephrine* is produced in, stored in, and released from tiny bubble-like *"vesicles"* in *sympathetic nerve terminals.* For *norepinephrine* to be produced in the *vesicles* requires another transporter, called the *"vesicular monoamine transporter,"* or *"VMAT."* A problem with any of these enzymes, co-factors, or the *VMAT* can result in decreased *norepinephrine* production and therefore low *plasma norepinephrine levels,* regardless of the rate of *sympathetic nerve traffic.*

Fourth, the *plasma norepinephrine level* usually is measured in a blood sample drawn from a vein in the arm. Because the skin and skeletal muscle in the forearm and hand contain many *sympathetic nerve terminals,* the *plasma norepinephrine level* in blood from an arm vein is determined not only by the amount of *norepinephrine* release from *sympathetic nerve terminals* in the body as a whole but also by the amount of release locally in the forearm and hand.

Fifth, the *plasma norepinephrine level* varies depending on the posture of the person at the time of blood sampling (the level doubles within minutes of standing up from lying down), the time of day (highest in the morning), whether the person has been fasting, the temperature of the room, dietary factors such as salt intake, and any of a large number of commonly used over-the-counter and prescription drugs or herbal remedies.

Plasma Epinephrine (Adrenaline) Levels

Compared to the *plasma norepinephrine level,* which is complexly and indirectly related to *sympathetic nervous system* "activity" in the body as a whole, the *plasma epinephrine (adrenaline) level* is a fairly direct indicator of activity of the *adrenomedullary hormonal system.*

> *Plasma epinephrine (adrenaline) is used to test the adrenomedullary hormonal system.*

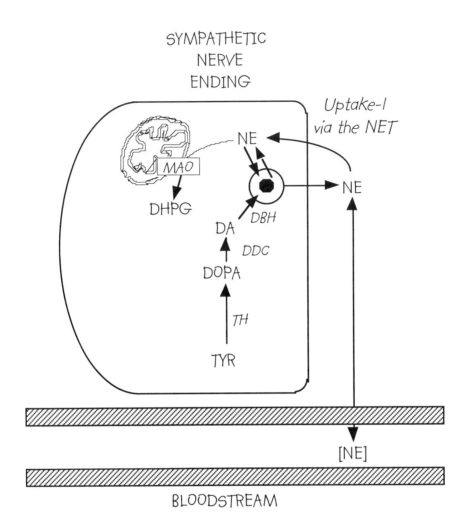

SYMPATHETIC
NERVE
ENDING

Uptake-1
via the NET

NE

MAO

DHPG

NE

DA   DBH

DDC

DOPA

TH

TYR

[NE]

BLOODSTREAM

Several factors influence plasma norepinephrine levels.

Nevertheless, some of the same factors that make interpreting *plasma norepinephrine levels* difficult can complicate interpreting *plasma epinephrine levels.* A large number of common and difficult to control life experiences that influence activity of the *adrenomedullary hormonal system.* These include drugs, alterations in blood *glucose* levels (such as after a meal), body temperature, posture, and emotional distress.

An additional problem is technical. *Epinephrine* is a very powerful *hormone.* Not surprisingly, the *plasma epinephrine level* normally is very low. The level can be so low that it is about at or below the limit of sensitivity of the measurement technique, which would invalidate the result. Other chemicals besides *epinephrine* can interfere with the measurement. This can especially be a problem in people who drink a lot of coffee, even if it is decaffeinated, because of high plasma levels of a chemical called *dihydrocaffeic acid,* which can mimic *epinephrine* in some assay procedures.
Because of these issues, it is important that blood sampling and chemical assays for *plasma epinephrine levels* be carried out by experienced and expert personnel.

Neuroimaging Tests

Compared to other types of testing for *dysautonomias,* testing using *neuroimaging* is new.

Neuroimaging is a way to actually see nervous system tissue, such as in the brain. In testing for *dysautonomias,* the neuroimaging involves seeing the *sympathetic nerves* in an organ outside the brain, such as in the heart.

Sympathetic nerves in the heart travel with the *coronary arteries* that deliver blood to the heart muscle. The nerves then dive into the muscle and form mesh-like networks that surround the heart muscle cells. Because *neuroimaging tests* have a limit of resolution of a few millimeters, the imaging does not show individual nerves but gives a general picture, and because the nerves are found throughout the heart muscle, the picture looks very much like a scan of the heart muscle.

The radioactive drugs used for imaging the *sympathetic nerves* in the heart are given by vein, and they are delivered to the heart muscle by way of the *coronary arteries.* This means that one must be able to distinguish a local loss of radioactivity in the scan that is due to loss of *sympathetic nerves* from a local loss that is due to a place where the *coronary artery* is blocked, because either nerve loss or coronary blockage could lead to the same lack of radioactivity in the heart muscle.Centers that carry out *sympathetic neuroimaging* therefore often do two scans in the same test, one scan to see where the blood is going and one to see where the *sympathetic nerves* are.

MIBG Scanning

In the United States, *sympathetic neuroimaging* is available in few centers but is available fairly widely in European countries and Japan. Worldwide, probably the most commonly used *sympathetic neuroimaging* agent is *123I-metaiodobenzylguanidine*, or *123I-MIBG*. *123I-MIBG* is a radioactive form of a drug that is taken up by sympathetic nerve terminals, making them visible on a nuclear medicine scanner.

Fluorodopamine PET Scanning

At the National Institutes of Health's Clinical Center, in Bethesda, Maryland, another *sympathetic neuroimaging* agent has been developed, which is *6-[18F]fluorodopamine*. This is a radioactive form of the *catecholamine, dopamine.* After injection of *6-*

[¹⁸F]fluorodopamine, by vein, the drug is taken up by sympathetic nerve terminals, and the radioactivity is detected by a special type of scanning procedure called *positron emission tomographic scanning,* or *"PET scanning."*

Imagine you had a radioactive object in a box. You could determine if there were something radioactive inside by using a detector, such as a Geiger counter. Now imagine that you had many little Geiger counters all around the box. Each counter would detect a different amount of radioactivity, depending on the shape of the object and the distance of the counter from the object. If you had a way to construct a picture, such as in a newspaper photo, where the size and intensity of each dot depended on the amount of radioactivity, then you could construct an image of the object inside the box. *Tomographic scans* are two-dimensional images, or slices. *Tomographic* slices would allow you to see what was inside the box at any level. If the object were small, most of the slices would be empty. Eventually, at the level of the object, you would see an image of the object in the slice.

A *positron* emitter is a type of radioactive substance that releases a short-lived form of radiation that can penetrate the body and reach detectors outside it, enabling construction of a *PET* scan. Other scans in nuclear medicine use a somewhat different source of radioactivity, but the idea is about the same.

Fluorodopamine is structurally similar to the biochemicals of the *sympathetic nervous system,* norepinephrine (noradrenaline) and epinephrine (adrenaline). Just as some radioactive chemicals get taken up by bone, producing a bone scan, or get taken up by the brain, producing a brain scan, fluorodopamine gets taken up by *sympathetic nerve endings,* and the result is a scan of the *sympathetic nervous system.* For instance, we know that *fluorodopamine* gets taken up very readily in the heart walls, since there are so many *sympathetic nerve endings* there. Because there are so many sympathetic nerve endings in the heart, *PET* scans of the heart after injection of *fluorodopamine* basically look like images of the heart itself. One can easily make out the main pumping muscle *(left ventricular myocardium),* the *septum* between the left and right *ventricles,* and the left and right ventricular chambers that contain the blood the heart pumps.

Different forms of *dysautonomia* result in remarkably different pictures of the *sympathetic nerves* in the heart by *fluorodopamine PET scanning.* Probably the most striking pictures occur in diseases where there is a loss of sympathetic nerve terminals, such as in *pure autonomic failure* and in *Parkinson's disease,* because even when the blood flow to the heart muscle is normal, there is no heart visible in the *PET scan!*

A much more difficult issue is whether analysis of the amount of radioactivity in the heart can provide information about how the *sympathetic nerve terminals* are functioning. This is a matter of research interest now.

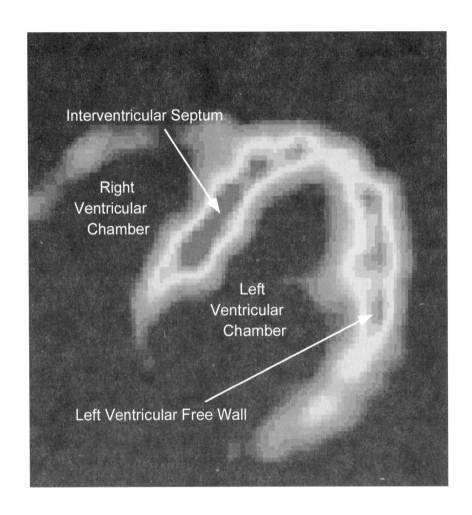

Fluorodopamine PET scanning can show the sympathetic nerves in the heart muscle.

Treatments for Dysautonomias

Successful treatment of *dysautonomias* usually requires an individualized program, which can change over time.

You should understand that since the underlying mechanisms often are not understood well, treatment is likely to involve some trial and error.

Non-Drug Treatments

Several non-drug treatments are used for different types of *dysautonomias*. The reasons for a treatment depend on the particular *dysautonomia*. Sometimes, the responses of a patient to a treatment help the doctor determine the diagnosis. Patients with *dysautonomias* can feel differently from day to day, even without any clear reason why.

This means that if a treatment is tried, it may take several days to decideon whether the treatment has helped or not.

Elevation of the Head of the Bed

In patients who have a fall in blood pressure every time they stand up *(orthostatic hypotension),* elevation of the head of the bed at night, by a variety of ways, improves the ability to tolerate standing up in the morning.

Salt Intake

High salt intake tends to increase the volume of fluid in the body. A small percent of this volume is in the bloodstream. Doctors usually recommend a high salt diet for patients with an inability to tolerate prolonged standing *(chronic orthostatic intolerance)* or a fall in blood pressure during standing *(orthostatic hypotension).* Normally when a person takes in a high salt diet, the kidneys increase the amount of salt in the urine, and this limits the increase in *blood volume.* Drugs that promote retention of *sodium* by the kidneys, such as *Florinef*™, are usually required for high salt intake to increase body fluid volume effectively.

Meals

Eating a big meal leads to shunting of blood toward the gut. In people with dizziness or lightheadedness when they stand up *(orthostatic intolerance)* or with *orthostatic hypotension,* it is usually advisable to take frequent small meals.

Reducing the amounts of sugars or other carbohydrates in meals may help manage symptoms.

Compression Hose

Compression hose or other compression garments tend to decrease the amount of pooling of blood in veins when a person stands. This can decrease leakage of fluid from the veins into the tissues and decrease swelling of the feet. In patients with veins that fill up or leak excessively during standing, compression garments can improve toleration of prolonged standing. In patients with a fall in blood pressure during standing (orthostatic hypotension), the problem may be less with the veins than with the arteries and arterioles, the blood vessels that carry oxygen-rich blood under high pressure to the organs and limbs. Wearing compression garments therefore may be disappointing in the management of orthostatic hypotension.

Coffee

Some patients with dysautonomias feel better drinking caffeinated coffee frequently. Others feel jittery or anxious and avoid caffeinated coffee. Still others notice no effect one way or the other.

Temperature

Patients with *dysautonomias* often have an inability to tolerate extremes of external temperature. When exposed to the heat, patients with failure of the *sympathetic nervous system* may not sweat adequately to maintain the core temperature by evaporation of the sweat. Patients with *chronic orthostatic intolerance,* such as from *postural tachycardia syndrome (POTS),* can have heat intolerance because of loss of blood volume by sweating or shunting of blood away from the brain. When exposed to cold, patients with *sympathetic nervous system* failure may not constrict blood vessels adequately in the skin, so that the body temperature falls *(hypothermia).*

Exercise

Patients with *dysautonomias* sometimes benefit from an exercise training program. Often, however, the training does not decrease the sense of fatigue.

As a person exercises, the blood vessels carrying oxygen-rich blood to the exercising muscle *(arteries and arterioles)* tend to relax, due at least partly to the accumulation of byproducts of metabolism. The *sympathetic nervous system* normally counters this tendency, by increasing the tone of the blood vessel walls. The blood flow to the exercising muscle therefore is in a dynamic state of balance. Activation of *sympathetic nerves* to the heart during exercise increases the force and rate of the heartbeat, and the total amount of blood pumped by the heart in one minute *(cardiac output)* increases. Meanwhile, like squeezing a tube of toothpaste, pumping of muscle during exercise increases the movement of blood from the limbs back to the heart. The increased metabolic activity tends to increase body temperature, and sweating, which is stimulated importantly by *sympathetic nerves* to sweat glands, increases the loss of heat by evaporation, helping maintain an appropriate body temperature.

If a patient had failure of the *sympathetic nervous system,* excessive production of byproducts of metabolism, or a form of heart disease where there were an inability to increase the force or rate of the heartbeat, then the blood pressure would fall during exercise, producing a sense of fatigue or exhaustion.

After exercise, when muscle pumping ceases, the blood can begin to pool in the legs or abdomen, while the rate of *sympathetic nerve traffic* falls to the resting rate. If the decline in *sympathetic nerve traffic* did not balance the decline in production of byproducts of metabolism, then the blood pressure would fall after exercise. At the same time, loss of body fluid via evaporative sweating would decrease the blood volume. Patients with a *dysautonomia* therefore can feel bad not only during exercise but also after exercise. It is important to stay hydrated and to avoid activities like eating a large meal after exercise, because this can divert already limited blood volume to the gut.

Perhaps surprisingly, even vigorously healthy, muscular, lean people can have a susceptibility to faint *(neurocardiogenic syncope),* and it is unclear if exercise training in general helps them. On the other hand, some patients can improve by isometric calf muscle training, where the patient learns to tense calf muscles when standing. This tends to decrease the amount of pooling of blood in the legs.

Pacemakers and Sinus Node Ablation

Insertion of a pacemaker in the heart can help patients with *neurocardiogenic syncope* or *POTS.* This is an area of active research and some controversy. In some patients with *neurocardiogenic syncope,* having a pacemaker inserted may not be a cure, because the low pulse rate at the time of fainting might not cause and might even be the result of low blood flow to the brain. On the other hand, a sudden absence of electrical activity in the heart produces loss of consciousness within seconds, and in this setting a pacemaker could be curative.

Some patients who have a very fast pulse rate undergo destruction of the *sinus node* pacemaker cells in the heart *(sinus node ablation)*. The doctor must be sure that the fast pulse rate results from a problem with the heart and does not result from a compensation by the *sympathetic nervous system* for another problem, such as low blood volume, because eliminating the compensation could make the patient worse rather than better.

Neurosurgery

Some patients with *chronic orthostatic intolerance* have a type of change in the brainstem called *Chiari malformation*. This is an anatomic abnormality where part of the brainstem falls below the hole in the skull between the brain and spinal cord. Neurosurgery can correct the malformation, but the *orthostatic intolerance* does not necessarily disappear. This is a controversial topic, and we recommend that patients seek a second opinion before agreeing to this procedure.

Constipation or Urinary Retention

Patients with failure of the *parasympathetic nervous system* can have problems with constipation and retention of urine in the bladder. The constipation is treated non-specifically, with stool softeners, bulk laxatives, and if needed milk of magnesia, magnesium citrate, senna, or cascara. Urinary retention can be associated with urinary urgency and incontinence. Drugs that stimulate *receptors* for *acetylcholine*, such as *urecholine,* might be tried.

Often patients with *autonomic failure* must learn to self-catheterize to empty the bladder, by inserting a plastic or rubber tube into the urethra and then into the bladder, in order to obtain relief.

Water Drinking

A relatively recently described tactic to increase blood pressure in patients with *autonomic failure* is to drink 16 ounces of water or other fluid. Why water drinking should increase blood pressure in patients with *autonomic failure,* when doing so does not affect the blood pressure of healthy people, remains unclear.

Patients with *chronic orthostatic intolerance, neurocardiogenic syncope,* or *POTS* often keep a water container with them and sip from it repeatedly during the day. This habit might indicate a tendency to dehydration and low blood volume, but the meaning of what we call the "water bottle sign" remains unproven.

Drug Treatments

Several drug treatments are used for *dysautonomias*. Some of them are powerful or can produce bad effects. Patients should take medications only under the supervision of a doctor with expertise and experience in the treatment of *dysautonomias*.

Fludrocortisone (Florinef™)

Florinef™ is a man-made type of drug called a *salt-retaining steroid,* or *mineralocorticoid. Florinef™* closely resembles the body's main *salt-retaining steroid,* which i*s aldosterone.*

Florinef™ must be taken with a high-salt diet to work. *Florinef™* forces the kidneys to retain *sodium,* in exchange for *potassium.* Water follows the sodium, and so *Florinef™* is thought to increase the blood volume. The patient gains "fluid weight," and blood pressure increases. Because of the tendency of *Florinef™* to waste *potassium, Florinef™* can cause a fall in the serum *potassium* level, which if severe can be dangerous. Patients taking *Florinef™* should have periodic checks of their serum *potassium* level, and if it is low take a *potassium* supplement.

Aldosterone

Fludrocortisone
(Florinef™)

> *Florinef™ forces the body to retain salt.*

Florinef™ given to patients with *chronic autonomic failure* can cause or worsen high blood pressure when the patient is lying down. Sometimes the doctor faces a difficult dilemma, balancing the long-term increased risk of stroke, heart failure, or kidney failure from high blood pressure against the immediate risk of fainting or falling from *orthostatic hypotension.*

Beta-Adrenoceptor Blockers

The main chemical messenger of the *sympathetic nervous system* is *norepinephrine (noradrenaline)* and of the *adrenomedullary hormonal system* is *epinephrine (adrenaline). Norepinephrine* and *epinephrine* produce their effects by binding to specific *receptors* on the target cells, such as heart muscle cells. There are two types of *receptors* for *norepinephrine* and *epinephrine,* called *alpha-adrenoceptors* and *beta-adrenoceptors.*

Epinephrine (adrenaline), which stimulates both *alpha-adrenoceptors* and *beta-adrenoceptors,* produces *vasoconstriction* in most parts of the body, such as the skin, due to stimulation of *alpha-adrenoceptors,* but with the important exception of the skeletal muscle, where the blood vessels relax, due to stimulation of *beta-adrenoceptors.* Because of the relaxation of the blood vessels in skeletal muscle, stimulation of *beta-adrenoceptors* tends to decrease the *total peripheral resistance.* Stimulation of *beta-adrenoceptors* also produces powerful effects on the heart, increasing the force and rate of the heartbeat. Because of the effects on the heart, the amount of blood pumped by the heart per minute *(cardiac output)* increases, and this increases the blood pressure when the heart is contracting, the *systolic blood pressure.*

There are at three types of *beta-adrenoceptors,* called beta-1, beta-2, and beta-3. *Beta-1 adrenoceptors* and *beta-2 adrenoceptors* are present in the human heart, and stimulation of these receptors produces about the same effects. In contrast, *beta-2 adrenoceptors* are much more abundant in skeletal muscle blood vessels than are *beta-1 adrenoceptors.* This difference may be relevant to the treatment of *neurocardiogenic syncope,* as explained below.

Beta-adrenoceptor blockers decrease the pulse rate, the force of heart contraction, and the *systolic blood pressure.* In patients with rapid pulse rates, associated with a sense of pounding or irregular beating of the heart *(palpitations)* or chest pain, *beta-adrenoceptor blockers* decrease the heart rate and can help relieve the pain and prevent abnormal heartbeats or heart rhythms; however, in patients where the chest pain results from stimulation of *alpha-adrenoceptors* in the *coronary arteries, beta-adrenoceptor blockers* may not help the pain. These drugs also are commonly used to treat long-term high blood pressure *(hypertension).* Because of decreased *systolic blood pressure* and heart rate, the rate of consumption of oxygen by the heart decreases, and this can help patients with *coronary artery disease.*

Non-Selective	Selective
Propranolol (Inderal™)	Atenolol (Tenormin™)
Nadolol (Corgard™)	Metoprolol (Toprol™)
Timolol (Blocadren™)	Betaxolol (Kerlone™)

> *Here are some beta-blockers. All beta-blockers decrease the rate and force of the heartbeat.*

In patients with *postural tachycardia syndrome (POTS)*, the value of treatment with *beta-adrenoceptor blockers* may depend on whether the rapid pulse rate when the patient stands up reflected a primary or compensatory response. If the rapid pulse rate were a compensation for another problem, such as low blood volume due to bleeding, then blocking that compensation would not help the patient. But if the rapid pulse rate were the result of an inappropriate, excessive rate of *sympathetic nerve traffic* to the heart, then blocking the effects of the excessive nerve traffic would help the patient.

There are two types of *beta-adrenoceptor blockers,* selective and non-selective. Selective *beta-adrenoceptor blockers* block beta-1 adrenoceptors, and non-selective *beta-adrenoceptor blockers* block both *beta-1 adrenoceptors* and *beta-2 adrenoceptors.* A potentially important difference between these drugs is that non-selective *beta-adrenoceptor blockers* block the *beta-2 adrenoceptors* in blood vessel walls of skeletal muscle, whereas *beta-1 adrenoceptor blockers* do not. In patients with *neurocardiogenic syncope* and high levels of *epinephrine* in the bloodstream, the *epinephrine* might stimulate *beta-2 adrenoceptors* on blood vessels in skeletal muscle. This would relax the blood vessels, decreasing the resistance to blood flow. This in turn could shunt blood away from the brain and towards the limbs, contributing to lightheadedness or loss of consciousness. In such patients, *non-selective beta-adrenoceptor blockers* might be preferable to selective blockers.

Midodrine (Proamatine™)

Midodrine (Proamatine™) is a relatively new drug that tightens blood vessels throughout the body. That is, it is a *vasoconstrictor. Midodrine* works by stimulating *alpha-adrenoceptors* in blood vessel walls.

Midodrine (Proamatine™) is used to treat conditions where there is a failure to tighten blood vessels appropriately, such as when a patient stands up. When a person stands up, the *sympathetic nervous system* is normally activated reflexively, the chemical messenger *norepinephrine* is released from the *sympathetic nerve terminals* in blood vessel walls, the *norepinephrine* binds to *alpha-adrenoceptors* in the blood vessel walls, and the stimulation of the *alpha-adrenoceptors* causes the blood vessels to constrict *(vasoconstriction),* increasing the blood pressure.

Midodrine acts like an artificial form of norepinephrine, by stimulating *alpha-adrenoceptors* directly. In some patients with a fall in blood pressure when they stand up *(orthostatic hypotension),* the cause is a loss of *sympathetic nerve terminals,* so that there is little or no *norepinephrine* to release. In this situation, the *alpha-adrenoceptors* on the cells in blood vessel walls accumulate on the cell surface, and the blood vessels become supersensitive *(denervation supersensitivity).* In these patients, *midodrine* can be very effective in raising the blood pressure.

In using *midodrine* to treat elderly men with *orthostatic hypotension,* the doctor should be aware that stimulation of *alpha-adrenoceptors* can worsen symptoms of prostate problems, such as urinary retention, urgency, and decreased urinary stream. *Alpha-1 adrenoceptor blockers* are effective in treating *benign prostatic hypertrophy (BPH),* and *alpha-1 adrenoceptors blockers* interfere with *midodrine.*

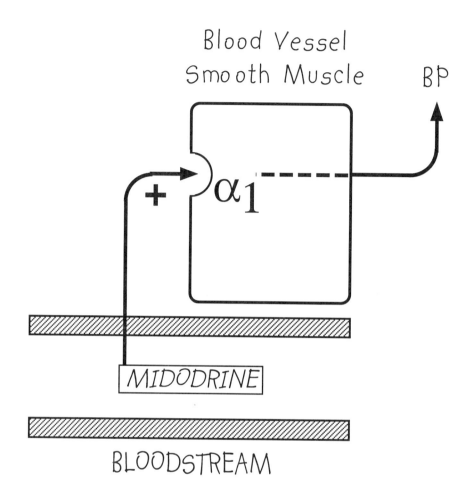

Blood Vessel
Smooth Muscle   BP

$+$ α_1

MIDODRINE

BLOODSTREAM

Midodrine works like artificial norepinephrine, increasing blood pressure (BP) by stimulating alpha-adrenoceptors in blood vessel walls.

Clonidine

There are two types of *alpha-adrenoceptors,* called alpha-1 and alpha-2. Stimulation of either type of *receptor* in blood vessel walls causes the vessels to constrict *(vasoconstriction).*

Clonidine stimulates *alpha-2 adrenoceptors.* Stimulation of *alpha-2 adrenoceptors* in the brain decreases the rate of *sympathetic nerve traffic.* Stimulation of *alpha-2 adrenoceptors* on *sympathetic nerve terminals* decreases the amount of release of the chemical messenger, *norepinephrine,* from the terminals. Therefore, even though *clonidine* stimulates a type of *alpha-adrenoceptor, clonidine* normally decreases blood pressure.

> *Clonidine works both in the brain and outside the brain. It decreases the blood pressure and often causes drowsiness.*

There are several uses of *clonidine* in the diagnosis and treatment of *dysautonomias.* In the *clonidine suppression test,* discussed in the section about tests for *dysautonomias, clonidine* is used to separate high blood pressure due to increased *sympathetic nervous system* activity from high blood pressure due to a tumor that produces *norepinephrine* and *epinephrine,* called *pheochromocytoma.* In patients with long-term high blood pressure *(hypertension)* due to excessive release of *norepinephrine* from *sympathetic nerve terminals (hypernoradrenergic hypertension), clonidine* can be very effective in lowering the blood pressure. Clonidine is also effective in treating withdrawal from some addictive drugs.

Clonidine usually causes drowsiness and often causes a dry mouth. The sedation from *clonidine* can limit its use.

Yohimbine

When *alpha-2 adrenoceptors* in the brain are blocked, this increases *sympathetic nerve traffic and* increases the amount of *norepinephrine* release for a given amount of *sympathetic nerve traffic.*

Yohimbine blocks *alpha-2 adrenoceptors* in the brain and on *sympathetic nerve terminals,* and so it releases *norepinephrine* from the terminals. The released norepinephrine binds to *alpha-1 adrenoceptors* in blood vessel walls. This causes the blood pressure to increase.

Even though *yohimbine* blocks *alpha-2 adrenoceptors* in blood vessel walls, the drug releases so much *norepinephrine,* and there are so many *alpha-1 adrenoceptors* in blood vessel walls, that normally *yohimbine* increases the *plasma norepinephrine level* and increases the *blood pressure.*

In patients with *chronic autonomic failure* and an inability to regulate *sympathetic nerve traffic* to intact

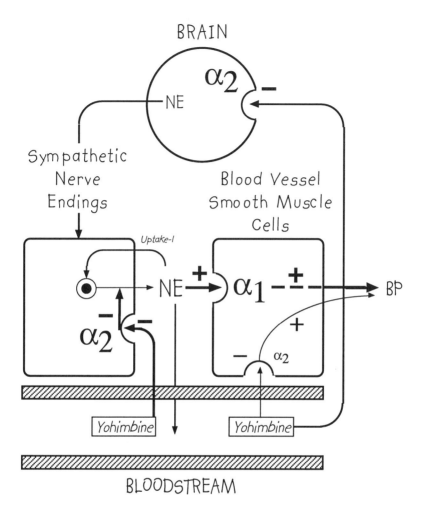

Yohimbine works both in the brain and outside the brain. The drug increases blood pressure and the state of alertness.

terminals, such as in the *Shy-Drager syndrome,* *yohimbine* releases *norepinephrine* from the terminals and effectively increases the blood pressure. In patients with *neurocardiogenic syncope, yohimbine* may prevent episodes of fainting.

Yohimbine can cause trembling, paleness of the skin, goosebumps, hair standing out, an increase in salivation, or emotional changes.

Oral *yohimbine* is approved as a prescription drug to treat impotence from *erectile dysfunction* in men. *Yohimbine,* in the form of *yohimbe bark,* can be purchased in health food stores.

Intravenous Saline

Inability to tolerate prolonged standing can result from low blood volume, excessive pooling of blood in the veins of the legs during standing, or exit of fluid from the blood vessels into the tissues during standing *(extravasation).* In these situations, infusion of physiological saline solution can temporarily improve the ability to tolerate standing up. This is also useful for diagnostic purposes. Some patients with *chronic orthostatic intolerance* benefit from intravenous saline infusion given repeatedly by way of a permanent intravenous catheter.

Amphetamines

Amphetamines are chemicals that resemble the drug, *dextro-amphetamine,* or *d-amphetamine.*

Amphetamines are in a class of drugs called *indirectly acting sympathomimetic amines.* They produce their effects at least partly by increasing delivery of *norepinephrine* to its *receptors,* both in the brain and outside the brain.

By way of effects in the brain, *amphetamines* increase the state of arousal and attention, prevent or reverse fatigue, decrease appetite, and at high doses increase the rate and depth of breathing. By way of effects on the *sympathetic nervous system,* they increase blood pressure.

Pseudephedrine (Sudafed™) is structurally a mirror image *(stereoisomer)* of *ephedrine.* This difference changes the properties of the drug, producing much less central nervous system stimulation. By releasing *norepinephrine* from *sympathetic nerve terminals* in the mucous membranes of the nasal airways, *pseudephedrine* tightens blood vessels, making them less leaky and thereby relieving nasal congestion.

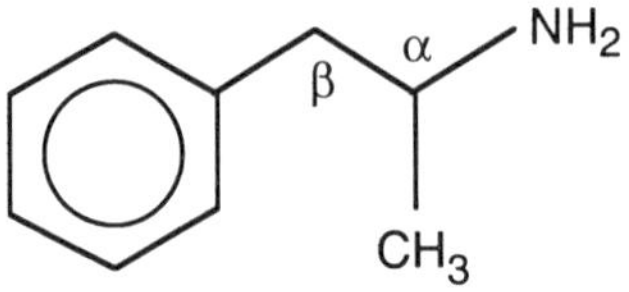

AMPHETAMINE

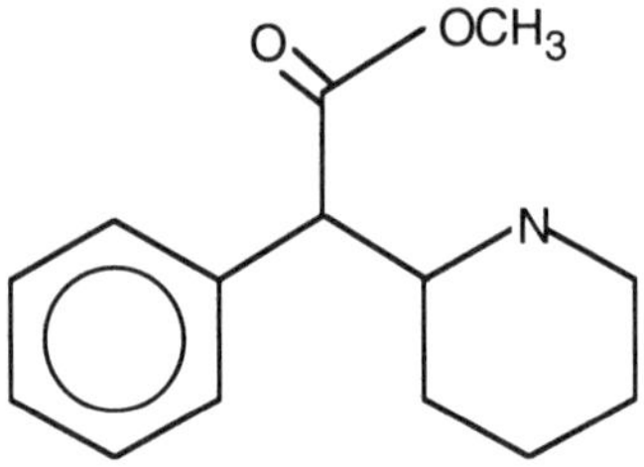

METHYLPHENIDATE

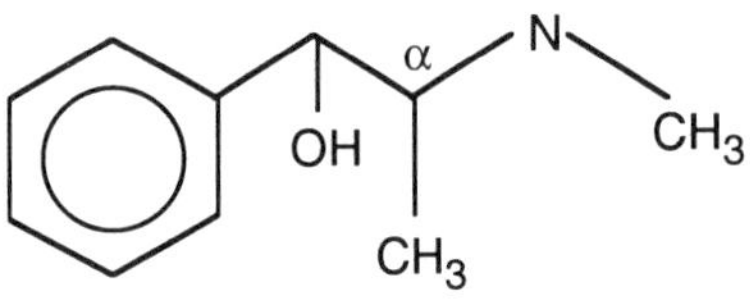

EPHEDRINE

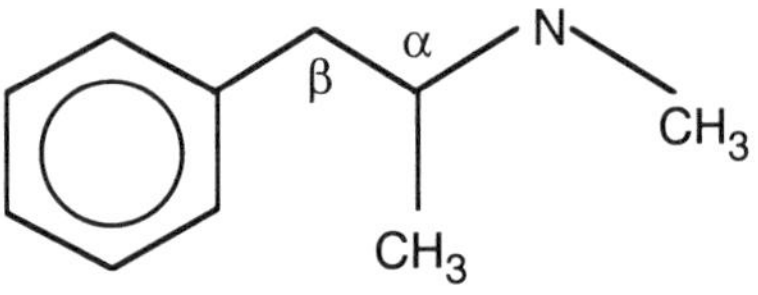

METHAMPHETAMINE

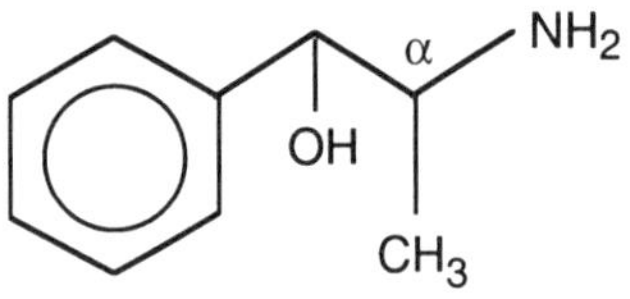

PHENYLPROPANOLAMINE

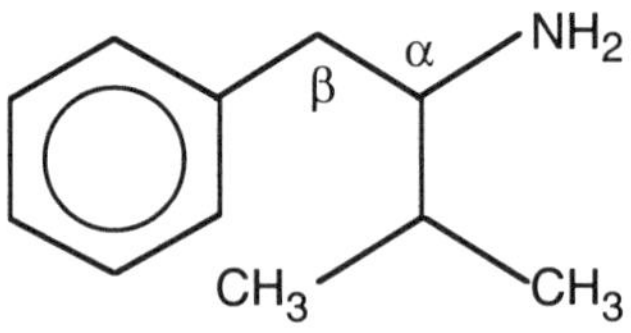

PHENTERMINE

Amphetamines work both inside and outside the brain. They increase attention, decrease appetite, interfere with sleep, and often increase the blood pressure.

Methylphenidate (Ritalin™), another *sympathomimetic amine*, is used commonly to treat attention deficit-hyperactivity disorder.

Phenylpropanolamine (PPE) until relatively recently was used in over-the-counter diet pills, until the discovery of serious adverse effects such as severe high blood pressure and stroke.

Phentermine prescribed with *fenfluramine ("Phen-Fen")* was an effective combination to decrease weight, until serious adverse effects of this combination came to light.

In treating patients with *dysautonomias, amphetamines* should be used sparingly, because of the potential for tolerance and dependence. In patients with *sympathetic neurocirculatory failure* from abnormal regulation of *sympathetic nerve traffic* to intact *sympathetic nerve terminals,* this type of drug releases *norepinephrine* from the terminals and increases the blood pressure. Some patients with *chronic orthostatic intolerance,* such as *neurocardiogenic syncope,* can improve.

Selective Serotonin Reuptake Inhibitors (SSRIs)

SSRIs inhibit a key process that is required for inactivating and recycling the chemical messenger, *serotonin*. The process is reuptake of released *serotonin* back into the nerve terminals that store it. *SSRIs* are widely used to treat depression, anxiety, and other psychiatric or emotional problems. They are also used to treat some forms of *dysautonomias.*

Procrit™ (Erythropoietin)

Procrit™ (Erythropoietin) is a particular hormone that is used as a drug. *Erythropoietin* in the body is released into the bloodstream by the kidneys and acts on the bone marrow to increase the production of red blood cells. *Procrit*™ therefore is helpful to treat low red blood cell counts *(anemia),* such as in kidney failure. Anemic patients look pale and feel tired. By mechanisms that remain incompletely understood, *Procrit*™ tends to increase the *blood pressure.* Some doctors prescribe *Procrit*™ to treat low *blood pressure* in patients with *chronic fatigue syndrome* who have a low red blood cell count.

L-Dihydroxyphenylserine (L-DOPS)

L-Dihydroxyphenylserine (L-DOPS) is a type of chemical called an *amino acid.* It is very closely related chemically to *L-dihydroxyphenylalanine (Levodopa, L-DOPA),* which is an effective drug to treat *Parkinson's disease. L-DOPA* works by being converted in the brain to the *catecholamine, dopamine. L-DOPS* works by being converted to the closely related *catecholamine, norepinephrine.* Since norepinephrine is the chemical messenger of the *sympathetic nervous system, L-DOPS* can provide *norepinephrine* even in the absence of *sympathetic nerve terminals.*

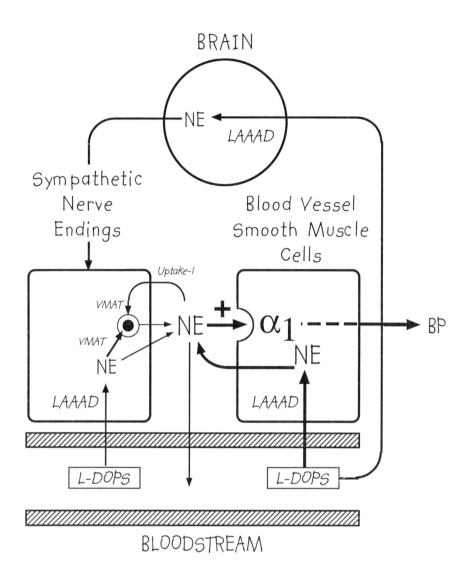

BRAIN

Sympathetic Nerve Endings

Blood Vessel Smooth Muscle Cells

BLOODSTREAM

L-DOPS is converted to norepinephrine both inside and outside the brain.

L-DOPS could increase delivery of *norepinephrine* to its *receptors* by at least three mechanisms. One is from uptake of *L-DOPS* into cells such as in blood vessel walls, followed by conversion of *L-DOPS* to *norepinephrine* that is speeded up by the enzyme, *L-aromatic-amino-acid decarboxylase (LAAAD)*. The *norepinephrine* exits the cells and binds to its *receptors* on the cell membrane. A second mechanism is from uptake of *L-DOPS* into *sympathetic nerve terminals,* again followed by conversion of *L-DOPS* to *norepinephrine.* The *norepinephrine* is taken up into storage *vesicles* and released in response to *sympathetic nerve traffic.* The *norepinephrine* exits the nerve terminals and binds to its *receptors* on cells in blood vessel walls. A third mechanism is from *L-DOPS* entering the brain, followed by conversion of *L-DOPS* to *norepinephrine.* The *norepinephrine* stimulates an increase in the rate of *sympathetic nerve traffic,* resulting in release of *norepinephrine* from the *sympathetic nerve terminals.* By all three mechanisms, *L-DOPS* administration would lead to stimulation of *alpha-adrenoceptors* in blood vessel walls, causing the vessels to constrict and increasing the blood pressure.

L-DOPS is currently an investigational drug. It has great promise to treat a fall in blood pressure when the patient stands up (*orthostatic hypotension)* or prevent fainting. A potential problem with using *L-DOPS* to treat *orthostatic hypotension* in patients with *Parkinson's disease* is that the patients often are treated at the same time with *Sinemet*™. *Sinemet*™ is a combination of *L-DOPA* and *carbidopa.* The *carbidopa* interferes with the conversion of *L-DOPA* to *dopamine.* Since *carbidopa* does not enter the brain, the combination results in increased delivery of *DOPA* to the brain and increased production of *dopamine. Carbidopa* also interferes with the conversion of *L-DOPS* to *norepinephrine.* This would be expected to prevent or blunt the hoped-for increase in blood pressure by *L-DOPS* treatment.

Bethanecol (Urecholine™)

Bethanecol is a drug that stimulates *receptors* for *acetylcholine,* the chemical messenger of the *parasympathetic nervous system.*

Urecholine™ increases production of saliva, increases gut activity, and increases urinary bladder tone.

Bethanecol increases the muscle tone of the bladder, digestive motions of the gut, and salivation. It may be useful to treat urinary retention or constipation in patients with *chronic autonomic failure,* but no formal study of this has been reported yet.

Drug	Goal of Treatment
Florinef™	Increase blood volume
=Fludrocortisone	Increase blood pressure
Proamatine™	Tighten blood vessels
=Midodrine	Increase blood pressure
	Prevent fainting
Beta-Blocker	Decrease heart rate
	Decrease blood pressure
	Decrease adrenaline effects
	Prevent fainting
Procrit™	Increase blood count
(=erythropoietin)	Increase blood pressure
Amphetamines	Tighten blood vessels
	Increase alertness
Desmopressin	Tighten blood vessels
"NSAID"	Tighten blood vessels
Octreotide	Tighten blood vessels in gut
SSRI	Improve mood, allay anxiety
"Tricyclic"	Improve mood
Xanax™	Increase sense of calmness
(=Alprazolam)	Improve sleep
Catapres™	Decrease blood pressure
(=Clonidine)	Improve sleep
Urecholine™	Increase salivation
(=Bethanecol)	Improve gut action
	Improve urination
Yohimbine	Increase blood pressure

> *Different centers use different drugs from a long "menu" to treat dysautonomias.*

Section B:
Living with
Dysautonomias

Living with Dysautonomias

Living successfully with a *dysautonomia* requires understanding how your body's "automatic nervous system" *(autonomic nervous system)* functions, and how changes in *autonomic nervous system* function may cause your symptoms. The first section of this book covers these topics. Living successfully with a *dysautonomia* also requires undertstanding how chronic illness impacts the patients, caregivers, and family, at home, at school, and at work—and requires important changes in lifestyle. This section of the manual gives you practical guidance for living successfully with *dysautonomias.*

Because causes of *dysautonomias* are not well understood, and because there are many forms of *dysautonomia,* your doctor and you will likely spend a lot of time trying to find reversible causes and devising a treatment program. For this reason, your relationship with your physician is crucial. We have included some suggestions on working with your doctor.

The changes that you and your family may face can place new emotional burdens on all members of the family. The following chapters include information on coping strategies, caregiving, finding or starting a support group, and the issue of children with a *dysautonomia*. Finally, having a chronic illness is likely to lead to inquiries about benefits that may be available from the insurance portion of Social Security. A summary of benefits is included, to help you understand your rights under this program.

Finding and Working with a Physician

Despite that fact that *dysautonomias* affect over a million Americans, you will probably find that very few people and even **few doctors have heard of *dysautonomias*.** It is likely that few if any doctors in your area specialize in treating autonomic disorders.

Few doctors have heard of dysautonomias.

Researchers over the last few years have brought to awareness the large number of people who are affected. Dr. David Robertson, of the Autonomic Dysfunction Center at Vanderbilt University, has called this awakening an ***"epidemic of disease recognition."*** With growing awareness, these disorders should become easier to recognize and treat.

It can be frustrating learning to live with a condition that others have never heard of, let alone try to pronounce (An easy way to remember it is to sound it out like this: **Dis** - like in <u>dis</u>tant, **auto** – like the car, **NO**- like what we tell our kids, **mia**- like Mia Farrow:

Dys—auto—NO-mia). The medical terminology can also be confusing. **The same basic set of symptoms can be called by a variety of names.** For example, symptoms of a long-term inability to tolerate standing up—*chronic orthostatic intolerance*—have been labeled as *"POTS" (Postural Orthostatic Tachycardia Syndrome,* or *Postural Tachycardia Syndrome), "COI" (Chronic Orthostatic Intolerance), Mitral Valve Prolapse-Dysautonomia Syndrome, Neurocirculatory Asthenia, Soldier's Heart, Neurally Mediated Hypotension,* and other names in a long list. It is no wonder that many patients feel frustrated and confused.

Finding a physician able to diagnose, treat, and follow your *dysautonomia* will likely take **effort on your part.** Unlike diseases or conditions that affect only one part of our body, *dysautonomias* can affect every part and system of our body. The *autonomic nervous system* plays a variety of roles in regulating many "automatic" functions, such as breathing, blood pressure, heart rate, digestion, sexual function, and other activities. Because of this, it is often difficult to determine which type of physician should manage the condition.

Your care may require some extra **effort by your doctor.** Since the cause of your symptoms may not be well understood, developing an effective treatment plan may take time. People with *dysautonomias* must be both patient and persistent. Because of large differences among patients, and continuing mystery about mechanisms of *dysautonomias,* doctors need to learn from their patients about what works and what doesn't.

Your first priority should be to **find a physician willing to work *with* you.** Whether that physician is a cardiologist, neurologist, endocrinologist, psychiatrist, internist, or family practitioner is less important than his or her ability to work with you and other physicians on your behalf.

Find a doctor who will work with you.

You and Your Doctor: A Working Relationship

Because little is known about underlying mechanisms of many forms of *dysautonomia*, **your physician will probably have the task of treating your symptoms without really knowing their exact cause.** For this reason, much of what will be done will be through a trial and error approach. Both you and your physician will need to have an understanding that finding a program that works will require time, patience, and open and honest communication. Your relationship and ability to communicate with your doctor will make a big difference in putting together an effective therapy program.

Your **symptoms are likely to change** over time. Keep your doctor informed about how you are doing and about changes you notice. For instance, a particular medication might make you feel better in one way but worse in another. Your doctor might be able to change your prescription or start you on another drug that would work the same way but with fewer side effects. If you notice major improvements, you should inform your doctor. It's possible you may not need as much medication to manage the problem.

Keep your doctor informed.

You should develop a plan with your doctor about **symptoms that require immediate attention** and those that can wait for a return visit. A brief discussion about this will help give you peace of mind when your symptoms are of concern.

Talking with a physician about multiple symptoms can be a problem, if you've had unpleasant interactions at office visits in the past. You might be concerned about what the doctor might think: "What if they think I'm CRAZY?" Don't let this concern keep you from relaying everything the doctor needs to know. You can't expect your physician to put the puzzle together if you keep out half the pieces. **Tell your physician about *all* your symptoms.** Let your doctor decide what is important information.

Create a bullet list of questions to ask. Many of us forget our questions unless we write them down. Keep in mind that your doctor has limited time to discuss your condition and treatment. Before visiting your doctor, ask yourself, "If I could improve one symptom, which would it be?" This type of thought process will give you and your physician a better opportunity to work on the symptoms that cause you the most trouble.

You may want to consider having a **family member or friend go with you.** Having someone with you may make you feel more comfortable, and a family member or friend can also give your physician details you may not recall.

Keeping a **daily journal** can also be a useful tool, both for you and your doctor. This may allow your doctor an opportunity to diagnose your condition and see trends or patterns in your symptoms. You might include blood pressure, pulse rate, body weight, and the timing and circumstances of events that trigger symptoms, mood, activity—even thoughts. Talk to your doctor about information to record. A one-month journal is usually adequate to give a picture. Let your doctor review your journal, since what may seem insignificant to you may be significant to your doctor. Keep in mind the nature of *dysautonomias,* in which symptoms often have peaks and valleys. Many women notice major changes while ovulating or having their period. You may notice changes if you become dehydrated, distressed, too warm, or even with a change in the weather. Keep track of your fluid and salt intake. Note whether resting in a recliner and reading a good book or magazine helps, and whether stimulation such as the radio, video games, or television makes a difference.

If your doctor starts you on a new medication, it is important to **discuss potential side effects**. You may want to purchase a reference source on prescription medication, such as the Family PDR. This manual lists the names of medications, their use, and side effects. It is helpful to know side effects triggered by your medication and not your condition.

Referral to an Autonomic Specialist

Physicians in several fields of medicine specialize in *dysautonomias.* Testing in a **specialized autonomic function testing laboratory** can help identify what form of autonomic involvement you have and speed development of an effective therapy program.

Consider specialized testing.

You should not feel reluctant to talk to your physician about going to another facility for testing. You will likely find that your physician will actually encourage you to visit one of these facilities, because the visit may provide valuable and otherwise unobtainable information that your doctor can use to help you.

Keep in mind that there are **relatively few autonomic function experts and testing laboratories.** For a list of physicians and facilities in your area, try visiting the website of the National Dysautonomia Research Foundation, www.ndrf.org, or give the Foundation a call at 651-267-0525.

Research Facilities – Should I Participate in a Study?

Many people who contact the NDRF ask about participation in research studies. There are a limited number of centers in the United States that conduct research on the *autonomic nervous system.* Patients are recruited to participate in these research studies, also known as "protocols". Each protocol has specific criteria for participation. For a list of ongoing studies you can contact the NDRF or visit the National Institutes of Health's Clinical Trial web site at: (www.clinicaltrials.gov).

Participation in a research study may help; however, it is important that you investigate the study thoroughly and review the consent information prior to participation.

Some **benefits of participating in research** are:

● You see physicians who specialize in this area of medicine. What may be unusual for your local physician may be routine for the physician conducting the research.

● You have the opportunity to learn more about what may be causing your symptoms. The testing could reveal important information about your condition that may not be available to your personal doctor.

● The medical institution typically covers the costs of the research testing, which otherwise would be expensive if available at all.

●	You help researchers understand the illness better, making it possible for them to devise sensible treatment plans and even look for new possible cures.

If you decide to participate in a study, keep in mind some of the possible **limitations of the research:**

●	You may be required to stop taking your medications, for the doctors to see how you function without them.

●	You may have to pay for travel.

●	Some tests can be painful, uncomfortable, or not directly related to your problem.

●	You may have to spend several days in the hospital.

●	You may need pre-certification from your insurance company. Testing at the research facility to confirm your diagnosis prior to the start of the study may have to be paid for through your medical insurance.

●	You have to meet the criteria for participation in the study. Not everyone qualifies, and research patients may not be recruited once a quota is filled.

●	Most important, you should understand that the usual primary focus of a research study is not to help a single patient but to learn more about the condition in general and how to treat it. Research studies therefore may not provide for long-term care or follow-up. This means that you will likely be returning to the care of your personal physician after participating in the research. Nevertheless, the researcher and the study results may help you and your doctor gain more knowledge about your condition and help devise an effective therapy program.

Physicians conducting research should not take the place of your local physician.

The research might give you immediate results, but alternatively it might take several months or even years before the research is completed and the results fully analyzed. You should have a clear understanding of what type of feedback to expect prior to your participation.

Keep educated about your condition. Passing along new information will help both you and your doctor. You will find that most physicians appreciate information provided them, especially if from a reliable source. Resource tools available today allow you a tremendous opportunity to stay abreast of new discoveries. You can find updates from a variety of sources, including the NDRF website, patient conferences, books, and newsletters. The National Library of Medicine's websites offer you easy access to medical search engines that can also help keep you informed of new research discoveries. Become your own advocate for improving your health!

Day by Day with Dysautonomia

This chapter stresses the importance of living with *dysautonomias* day by day. We thank Dr. Lisa Benrud-Larson, of the Mayo Clinic in Rochester, Minnesota, for her assistance.

Much of the information in this chapter comes from two sources; both are wonderful resources for individuals trying to learn how to cope with a chronic medical condition:

● *Taking Charge: How to Master the Eight Most Common Fears of Long-Term Illness.* Pollin R, Golant SK. Random House, 1994.

● *Living Well with a Hidden Disability.* Taylor S, Epstein R. New Harbinger Publications, Inc., 1999.

Additional material on chronic illness can also be found at the Mayo Clinic Internet site: *http://mayoclinic.com*

Chronic Illnesses

We are all familiar with acute illnesses such as the flu, strep throat, and pneumonia. They are generally treatable, have an identifiable cause, last a relatively short time, and involve a return to normal health.

In contrast, chronic illnesses, such as *dysautonomias,* chronic pain, or diabetes, can continue indefinitely. Their course can be affected by multiple factors, including heredity, environment, and lifestyle. Consequently, living with a chronic illness can be a continuous challenge, marked by many ups, downs, and unexpected turns.

> *Living with a chronic illness is a continuous challenge.*

Accepting Your Disorder

With an acute illness, you know you eventually will feel normal again. When you have a chronic illness, there often is no cure in the traditional sense. You may never return to your "normal" way of life. Adaptation and acceptance therefore become important in maintaining your quality of life.

The first step to accepting your condition is to understand it. Knowing the "details" (e.g., common symptoms) can alleviate uncertainty and help you learn how to manage life with a *dysautonomia.* Your physician or health care provider and the NDRF can help you with this.

> *Understand your condition.*

As suggested earlier, a daily journal can be extremely helpful, giving you get a better idea of your day-to-day experiences.

Modifying Your Life

Coping successfully with a chronic illness requires significant lifestyle changes. Modifying your lifestyle to help you maintain as "normal" a life as possible can help you gain a sense of control over your illness, rather than feeling your illness controls you.

Pacing your activities is very important. You might have been able to work 8 hours and then do chores at home, and now doing so would put you in bed for a week! You need to learn how to pace your activities, take "baby steps."

Making a **weekly chart of activities/tasks** that need to be done can help. Seeing things in black and white often helps in many ways. You might believe that you are not doing anything, yet when you actually make a list of your day-to-day activities, you may see you are trying to accomplish a great deal in one day or one week. The list can help you set priorities about tasks that definitely need to be accomplished that day or can be put off or eliminated.

It can also help in decisions about how responsibility for certain tasks might be shared among family members. For example, your spouse might take over the grocery shopping, or you might do only one load of laundry on a particular day. Deciding on the right balance between overdoing it and doing too little is not an easy task. It will take time and a lot of trial and error.

Do things you enjoy. This can distract you from your illness. Focus on hobbies and activities you can still do and look for new ones to replace those you no longer can pursue. An example would be avoiding a noisy art show outdoors in the heat and instead visiting an art museum in the cool indoors.

Know your limitations. Substituting one activity for another may become necessary in maintaining a sense of well-being. For instance, instead of scuba diving, which is strenuous physically, you could try snorkeling.

Our son plays little league baseball. Recently he asked if I could go to his game. As much as I wanted to be there to show support, I knew that going wasn't the brightest idea. So we improvised – my husband took the camcorder and taped it. This allowed us to watch it as a family - indoors where it is cool, and where I could watch a few minutes at a time. Not to mention it allowed our son an opportunity to see where he could strengthen his game!

Take an inventory of your interests. People often forget about things they had an interest in but have not thought about for years. Maybe you loved to paint as a high school student. This may be a good opportunity to get back into it.

Daily Life Tactics

There are several **basic tips** to pace your life:
- Get adequate rest
- Eat and drink right.
- Try to keep a regular schedule.
- Get an appropriate amount of exercise, as prescribed by your physician.
- Don't get dehydrated.
- Stay on your medication routine.

Mornings can be a very rough time. Start slowly and use your knowledge to help give yourself an edge. A study showed that patients who drink water before getting out of bed in the morning did better than patients who did not drink water. If your physician has advised you to increase both fluids and salt, a glass of V8 or tomato juice might be even more helpful, as these drinks contain large amounts of sodium.

Exercise plays an important role in treating most chronic conditions, including *dysautonomias*. Staying in shape improves your sense of well-being.

The veins in the legs contain one-way valves that allow blood to flow towards your heart without allowing it to back up into the legs. Muscle surrounds deep veins in the legs and compresses these veins when you contract your leg muscles. **Muscle pumping** helps to keep blood moving towards the heart and upper body when we stand upright. You can do different types of exercise to assist your venous pump. A very simple routine such as flexing your feet with one or two pound ankle weights will get the pump going. You can also tighten your calf, thigh, and buttocks muscles. Talk to your physician about whether muscle pumping would be right for you.

Showering If you suffer from lightheadedness when you stand up *(orthostatic intolerance),* you might feel worse taking a hot shower in the morning. Many patients with *chronic orthostatic intolerance* have heat intolerance. Consider taking your shower prior to going to bed at night.

Treatment for Anxiety or Depression Chronic illness, and especially chronic illness from an abnormality of the function of the *autonomic nervous system,* can increase the susceptibility to anxiety, panic, and depression. There is nothing wrong with asking your doctor if you might benefit from a medication to help you cope.

Avoid triggers that worsen your condition. Some triggers to keep in mind are:
●   Hot environment (e.g., hot shower, sauna, jacuzzi)

- *Dehydration* (not getting enough fluids)
- Emotional *distress*
- "Over-stimulation" (i.e., amusement parks, concerts, sporting events, video games)
- Large meals
- Alcohol
- Skipping medications

A ringing of a telephone can cause a "fight-or-flight" response. Turn the volume down!

Diet

Eating large meals tends to shunt blood toward the gut. This can also worsen *orthostatic intolerance* and make any *dysautonomia* patient feel sluggish, tired, and worn out, because less blood is delivered to the brain, heart and lungs. Try eating smaller meals, more often. A half bagel or English muffin or a small piece of fruit is a good way to start off the day. Sugary or starchy foods may also tend to make you more symptomatic.

During eating, you might try elevating your feet to heart level and exercise your legs, to keep the blood from pooling. Just flexing your feet back and forth can have a tremendous benefit.

The subject of what we eat is also very important. For many patients with *dysautonomias,* a diet high in salt and fluids is necessary, to maintain adequate blood pressure during standing. A half-cup of Campbell's chicken noodle soup has 890 mg of sodium. You should discuss salt intake with your doctor.

You might try avoiding foods high in sugar and starch. Some researchers have found that consumption of these substances can worsen symptoms. This is another matter to discuss with your doctor.

Environmental Temperature

Patients with *dysautonomia* can have intolerance to heat or cold. Our bodies have a built-in thermostat, and the *autonomic nervous system* is a key system the brain uses to regulate body temperature. It is therefore important to dress appropriately, as well as regulate the amount of time you expose yourself to heat or cold.

If you have heat intolerance and plan on being outdoors during the summer months, dress in cool and light clothes and remember to limit the amount of time you spend in the heat. Sitting under a tree might help to reduce the likelihood of heat exhaustion and yet still give you a chance to enjoy the outdoors. And force yourself to drink fluids.

Don't assume that your body has the capacity to warm itself when you are exposed to cold. Shivering is a natural response that our bodies have to keep warm. Just like sweating is a way to keep our body cool in the heat, shivering is a way the body stays warm in the cold. The nice thing about the cooler weather is the fact that you can always put on multiple layers, and cuddle up with a warm blanket. Electric blankets during the cold winter months are wonderful. Setting the blanket on low 15 minutes before getting into bed will avoid the shock of getting into an ice-cold bed.

Compression Stockings/Abdominal Compression

Compression stockings can help those of us who suffer from blood pooling in the lower half of the body, due to a problem with the veins. If you do use compression stockings, it can take some time to take them on and off. You may find it easier to put your stockings on and off while lying in bed. Lying down will keep you from becoming symptomatic while taking them off! It's also helpful to use a small amount of baby power when putting them on. Compression stockings may be ineffective in preventing a fall in blood pressure standing, when the problem is an inability to constrict *arterioles*.

L'eggs makes a line of affordable pantyhose for people with varicose veins. I purchased two pairs one size smaller than what I would normally wear, and wore both of them at the same time. I found them to be fairly comfortable, and easy to take on and off. Keep in mind however that they do not last as long as the compression stockings. If you wear stockings only occasionally, this may be an effective and less expensive approach to take. Abdominal compression has also been used to help treat pooling. Again wearing a girdle one size smaller than what you are can make a tremendous difference in how you feel. The combination of girdle and stockings can work well together. If wearing girdles or compression stockings isn't your style, try wearing bicycle pants.

Medic-Alert Bracelets

We recommend that patients with *dysautonomias* wear a Medic-Alert bracelet. This will speak on our behalf when we may not be in a position to speak for ourselves. The back of the bracelet can state "See wallet." Inside the wallet would be a piece of paper or laminated card about the condition, allergies and sensitivities to medications, names and phone numbers of physicians, and spouse or friend contact information. For information on obtaining a Medic-Alert bracelet, please visit their web site at http://www.medicalert.com/ or call 888-633-4298.

Work

Whether or not you keep working is an individual decision affected by a number of different factors (e.g., severity of symptoms, type of work, financial situation). There are no straightforward rules here.

> *It is likely your ability to work will be affected in some way by your illness.*

It may be that you can no longer put in 10-hour days. Perhaps you can no longer travel as part of your job. Maybe your job requires you to be on your feet all day, and that is just not possible any more.

If you want to continue to work, you might have to struggle with what, if anything, to tell your employer. Do you maintain your privacy, or let your employer know, so special accommodations can be arranged? This is a personal decision with no universal right or wrong answer. It may help to make a list of the pros and cons of disclosing your condition. Many things are going to affect your decision, including your specific work environment and job duties.

Work can involve episodes of emotional distress in healthy people, so it's no surprise that it can worsen physical symptoms in someone with a chronic illness. Just as you are going to have to make several lifestyle changes at home to manage your condition successfully, you're probably going to have to make changes at work. This might mean setting more limits. Where you used to skip that morning break and eat lunch at your desk, you may now need to take full advantage of the respite.

It can be scary and frustrating to have to "slow down" at work. You might be afraid of what will happen and what people will think of you. You have to remember that if you don't slow down, you may be jeopardizing your health, which in the long run will result in being able to do even less.

There may be a time when you have to discontinue working altogether. The decision to leave the work world, whether temporarily or permanently, can be accompanied by a whole host of emotions, including anxiety, depression, guilt, or relief.

To minimize anxiety associated with leaving work, structure your day (e.g., read books, listen to music, take a course over the internet, talk with friends), and try to learn something new. Maybe check out a library book on sketching or sewing. Make a list of your positive traits, to help remind you that you are of value even if you're not working.

If you are contemplating taking time off from work, be sure to investigate all your options regarding possible assistance. See the section about the Family and Medical Leave Act and disability leave.

Travel

Driving is one of the most important aspects of our independence and a necessity in everyday life. Faced with the reality that driving may cause risk not only to ourselves but to others, we must ask ourselves, "Is it safe for me to drive?" Discuss driving with your doctor. Your doctor can help to determine if your condition puts you at risk. If you are not able to continue driving, you will have to find ways others can help with your travel needs. Besides family, friends, and neighbors, your community may have programs. Your local chamber of commerce or United Way can give you information about public transportation and other programs.

Wearing **sunglasses** when you travel can reduce stimulus overload. You may notice that your symptoms don't seem as intense when you travel in the evening than in the daytime. Wearing earplugs can also help reduce the impact.

Wear a **girdle or compression stockings** while traveling. Abdominal compression helps us to keep blood from pooling to the feet, legs and stomach. Have you ever noticed a change in your skin color when you stand upright? You may notice that your feet and legs change to a purplish/blue! Compression garments will help you to keep the blood in the upper extremities where it belongs.

For many patients with *dysautonomias,* **air travel** can be a nightmare. Should you fly? Again it's always best to discuss this with your physician. If your physician tells you it is all right for you to fly, discuss the following to see if they make sense for you:

● Drink extra fluids for at least a couple of days before departure.
● Eat a diet high in salt (chips, pretzels, beef jerky, pickles).
● Avoid stressful, stimulating situations the day before or of departure. For instance, avoid going to the mall for last-minute shopping.
● Wear compression stockings and an abdominal compression garment.
● Wear earplugs.
● Take a couple deep breaths before takeoff.

- Ask your doctor about a medication to calm you and enable you to sleep during the flight.
- Fly with someone who knows your disorder. This will help if you have problems during the flight.
- Request bulkhead seating, so you can elevate your feet to heart level during the flight.
- Request a wheelchair at your destination.
- Try to arrange a day of rest after your flight.

When to Ask for Help

It is not easy to find the right balance between independence and help. You may need assistance in a variety of areas. At different points, you may need practical, financial, emotional, or physical help. Asking for help is more difficult for some than for others.

> *We all need help from others, whether we're healthy or not.*

People often feel guilty asking for help from family and friends. It might help to think about how things would be if the shoe were on the other foot. If your spouse or best friend had a chronic illness that required your assistance, would you resent a plea for help? Not likely!

Explaining exactly how someone can help can provide a sense of relief to the helper, who may not know what to do. You can make a list of the areas where you do and do not need assistance.

Don't assume that others can read your mind. You need to be clear in relating how you feel and what you need. Your friends, family, and caregivers need to do the same. This is not easy! You may not be sure of what you want. You may be afraid that you are asking too much or becoming a burden.

Social Activities

Staying involved in family and social activities as much as possible can help you cope with your illness. If you notice that these activities make your symptoms worse, then limit the time you spend on them. An example is a family picnic. If it is an all day function, plan on spending only an hour or two.

How do you tell your friends and family? How can you help them understand what you are going through? Obviously, you do not experience your illness in a vacuum. Those close to you are also significantly affected by your condition. They won't experience the same physical effects you do, but they will share other struggles (e.g., emotional, financial). This is a time of heightened stress and anxiety for the entire family.

Try to arrange a quiet time to sit down and talk with your family about issues related to your health. Explain clearly and speak directly. Ask if they understand what you're trying to say, and clarify what is not clear. Listen to what they have to say. Try to express yourself in a nonthreatening manner. Statements like *"Why do you always avoid me?"* will probably make your loved ones feel attacked and cause them to become defensive. Instead, try to phrase your statement in more neutral terms, such as, "Help me understand what you are going through. I feel like you don't want to be around me anymore and that hurts me. I miss being around you."

It is also important to give your loved ones permission for them to have their feelings. They are likely experiencing some of the same emotions you are, including anxiety and guilt. Anger and other negative emotions are also likely and normal. You and your family members can expect to feel hurt at times. Try to remember that these negative emotions are reactions to the situation and not to you yourself.

Trying to have a social life when you suffer from a *dysautonomia* can be a real challenge. People typically don't like to hear about others aches and pains, or how poor health prohibits participating in social events, such as going to church, parties, movies, sporting events, or school functions.

Attitude is Everything

It is easy to take a defeatist attitude and give up. It is natural to have negative thoughts when your world seems to be crashing in around you. People with chronic medical conditions are susceptible to experience increased emotional distress, fear, depression, anger, frustration, anxiety, or other negative emotions.

Even if you lack the physical capacity you had before becoming ill, you still have mental capacity. Consider Christopher Reeve. His paralysis didn't force him to give up. Instead he took his condition and gave the general public a look at the limitations that paralysis gives and turned it into an opportunity to help others who suffer from spinal cord injuries.

Lance Armstrong illustrates the power of determination and persistence. He was diagnosed with an advanced form of cancer that had already spread through his lungs, abdomen, and brain. He underwent extensive chemotherapy and several surgeries. Against all odds, he returned to the world of cycling and has won the Tour de France—repeatedly!

Some physical abnormalities in patients with a *dysautonomia* can themselves trigger mood swings. For instance, in several forms of *dysautonomia,* the blood pressure is extremely low when the patient stands up. This can evoke confusion, anxiety, or fear, due to decreased delivery of blood to the brain. In fact, mood swings can be a first indication of low blood flow to the brain. This may be a sign for you to increase your fluid intake. Remember it's wise to discuss changes in your mood, blood pressure, and other symptoms with your doctor.

Talking to others with the same condition can help. Even though we may not all have the same symptoms, we all have one thing in common—*dysautonomia* has changed our lives! There is nothing wrong with discussing your anger, frustration, concerns, and fears. A health psychologist may help you learn coping strategies. Some psychologists impress the importance of a "family session," where all members of the family can relate the effects that the illness has had on them. Keep in mind that the entire family is going to be impacted by your illness. Support groups can also be very helpful. Among other benefits, joining a support group helps you feel less alone.

Take time to **recognize your abilities** and what you *can* do. For example, you may need help with grocery shopping but not with putting the groceries away. It may take time to discover what you can still do despite your limitations. Make small goals. Your goal today might be to walk from the bedroom to the kitchen. Next month it might be to clean the kitchen.

Keeping a positive attitude will help you move on with your life. You must meet your challenges with determination. Blaming or attacking your physician, family, friends, or even God isn't going to improve your health. Having a positive attitude may! A positive attitude can result in faster recovery from surgery and burns, give patients more resistance to arthritis and cancer, and help improve immune function. Remember that those around you will also be affected by your illness. Your positive attitude will make things easier on your family, friends, neighbors, and yourself.

Caregiving

We thank David Levy for writing this chapter.

The chapter is divided into smaller sections: What is family caregiving? Who are family caregivers? What are their responsibilities? Why is family caregiving with *dysautonomias* so hard?

Dysautonomias, like few other chronic illnesses, can affect not only elderly people but also people under 40—especially women. Family caregiving in these circumstances becomes virtually unique. Rarely do you have kids as caregivers and the amount of young men as spousal caregivers for one illness.

Family Caregiving

Family caregiving is the act of taking care of and feeling responsible for another person, loved one or family member. It is not child rearing. It is more than being a husband or a wife. It is more than being a brother or sister. Caregiving has many faces and ages, with each situation a little different.

A Family caregiver is one who feels primary responsibility for the well-being of another family member experiencing limitations as the result of a chronic disease, injury, or illness. The spectrum of caregiving responsibilities and capabilities to create quality-of-life and well-being for another may entail emotional, physical, social, practical, financial, logistical, and psychological care and support.

It is difficult to identify caregivers, because they don't feel like caregivers. Much of what caregivers do is out of love, respect, and being "family." However, the emotional and practical wear and tear on caregivers is well documented and needs to be understood as a unique role. Love may be the motivation, but it clearly doesn't come with a set of instructions for long-term caregiving and can feel like a trap after months or years. Without understanding the responsibilities of family caregiver, many succumb to the anger, resentment, confusion, and physical ailments associated with long-term family caregiving.

While there is a lot to understand, much can be done. This is a family issue, which affects everyone in the family. Therefore, first and foremost is the need to **recognize the role of being a caregiver.** Not recognizing the caregiver role inherently prevents one from getting the understanding, help, support, and resources caregiver's needs.

Once the caregiver role is acknowledged, what happens next? Remember, we said love doesn't come with a set of caregiver instructions. Why caregiving is so hard?

● Because family caregiving involves the routine and repetitive, the day-to-day, psychological and social issues, economics and perhaps physical care needs, and the ongoing balancing act of work, household and other activities.

● Because it is not intuitive. Your maternal/paternal instincts and childrearing experience is not substitute training for what family caregivers must deal with. We do not have a "caregiver gene" in our DNA that blossom forth when we are confronted with these issues—like new mothers and bonding hormones. Ask yourself, "What training have I had in caregiving for a chronic illness?" Probably none, and the issue goes well beyond medical or nursing activities.

● Because there are lots of role reversals – kids caring for kids or parents; parents caring for each other and so on.

● Because we wait for a crisis rather than use long-term planning.

● Because family caregivers "burnt out" and feel that they are transparent, that everyone is focused on the care receiver, but no one recognizes the effort by the caregiver. Family caregivers can feel lonely, like they are in this by themselves and that no one understands what they are going through.

● Because no one has helped to manage the expectations of what the caregiver and care recipient are going to be facing.

If caregiving is not intuitive, it should come as no surprise that people don't know what they don't know. With no instructions; no planning and no clear understanding of the caregiver role the ongoing problems get harder to solve, not easier. If you don't take a hard look at what you are dealing with you are destined for difficulty. Expectation management is a key ingredient in being a successful caregiver. If you don't balance the long term hopes and dreams with the long-term realities its tough to plan and not be disappointed.

Caregiving for a dysautonomia patient is special.

Why is caregiving for someone with a dysautonomia different?

● You don't look sick. *Dysautonomia* caregiving is further complicated because the majority of people with *Dysautonomia* don't look like they're sick. Family, doctors, friends, schoolmates and relatives have a hard time believing in the illness. It raises questions of malingering, psychosomatic illness, and "being lazy" as well as the underlying issue of whether the caregiver is being manipulated. If the illness came with wheelchairs, leg braces, crutches and a limp everyone would line up to help.

● It isn't always short term. *Dysautonomia* can affect anyone at any age. It can strike people in their twenties, fifties, nineties and for some it can strike at birth! A chronic illness or disability such as congestive heart failure or stroke in an older person typically means 5-7 years of caregiving. With some forms of *dysautonomia* we may be talking about almost an entire lifetime, when the onset is at birth or during adolescence. The younger the individual when illness strikes, the greater the scope of impact. We are talking about lots of things being different: school, social life, relationships, future goals, responsibilities, intimacy, work issues, and the entire family structure.

Children as Caregivers

Whoever thought of **kids as caregivers**? It's true, especially with *dysautonomia.* Thousands of kids are helping to take care of their brothers and sisters and are living with the same feelings as grown-up caregivers. Kids are caregivers, because mom or dad has a chronic problem, and they are the ones at home. Kids don't think of themselves as caregivers, and they may be frightened by the confused feelings they have.

Most doctors and teachers never think about kids in this sort of role. Many parents never consider their kids as caregivers, but children as caregivers need to be recognized and supported for the valuable role they play.

Kids are the victims of stereotypes. No one considers them in the role of adults. If your children have this role, they need special support and a trusted outsider to talk to as well as Mom or Dad! Difficult stuff, but very real, and you can't keep your frustrations and confusion bundled up inside.

NDRF has a Kids Newsletter at the NDRF Website (www.ndrf.org). It's a great place to start.

Spousal Caregiving by Men

Spousal caregiving by men can be difficult, because men are not nurturers. Historically and culturally, men expect their home-based needs to be *met*, rather than being responsible for them. In male caregiving, social and business needs are curtailed or abbreviated to accommodate the spouse.

Men see themselves as the providers and defenders of hearth and community. To see a wife or partner suffering and feeling helpless or inadequate to relieve the pain and confusion create a sense of impotency in the protector.

Sexual and other shared pleasures may be limited or lost, leaving the husband feeling lonely and unappreciated.

Lost opportunities for promotion, business travel, or increased responsibility add to the burden. The potential alteration or dissolution of plans and dreams, expectations of life imposed upon by chronic issues must be faced. The lost opportunity of an anticipated future must be grieved. The process of grieving goes through stages from denial to acceptance and may last for years. Both partners may be grieving and need each others support, yet they may be at different stages on the road to acceptance.

Everyday life must be rearranged to accommodate the new reality and new plans laid or imposed. A new commitment must be made based on new understanding. Unresolved issues from the past with family (uncaring in-laws or parents) or with spouse (marital/sexual) may now be overwhelming. The role of spousal caregiver may not always be possible. Inevitably some will leave.
Often, however, one may find great courage, strength and renewed love in this long-term commitment to stay in the relationship

Intimacy

Intimacy is important in a normal relationship. It is very important in a relationship affected by caregiving, but is greatly impacted and strained by the limitations of the illness and the roles.

> *Intimacy is a major issue in caring for a spouse with a dysautonomia.*

You can love someone and never be intimate or sexual with him or her. You can have sex and never have intimacy with, or love for, the other person. You can love someone and have great intimacy without having physical sex. Whatever works for you is fine. If none of it works for you, or only in a limited way, you need to ask yourselves, Is it the illness? Is it the relationship? Is it blind acceptance of the "same old same old" and the anger of not doing anything about it? Whatever the reason, the subject of intimacy is at the core of many of the issues young couples face; it is inescapable for those dealing with chronic illness.

Sex is also a challenge. With *dysautonomia* you look fine, but feel awful. When you feel lousy, you don't feel sexy. That's a real strain on any marriage or relationship. Also, having a low libido can be a problem with many people who suffer with *dysautonomia* and their caregivers.

Your Are Not Alone

Whatever your beliefs, or whether you have a formal religion, having a sense of **spirituality**, an awareness of a greater force can be a tremendous comfort. Recent surveys of caregivers indicate that one of the best coping mechanisms is their spirituality and belief in a higher power. Use this as it fits for you. Derive the comfort it can bring.

If you really want to make your relationship work, you need inside and outside **professional help**– seek it. *Dysautonomia,* caregiving and the disruption to the family unit as well as the issues of money, disability, roles, childcare, and planning for the future bring myriad challenges.

The hope of this chapter is that if you are a family caregiver you will recognize **you are not alone.** Others have worked through similar life-changing events, and there is a positive future. You must recognize your problems and actively seek your own help. No one else is automatically coming to solve them for you.

Major organizations with family caregiver support, like the NDRF, create an opportunity for defining roles, outlining responsibilities, sharing information, and gaining better understanding. Just as important as knowing what doctor to go to and what medication to try is to recognize the major burden of family caregiving, but with the knowledge that you are not alone. Understanding this is not only helpful to those with chronic caregiving responsibilities, but their spouses, children, friends, and other family members as well.

Support Groups

We thank Suzette G. Levy for writing this chapter.

Support groups are an invaluable tool to helping others and oneself deal with the consequences of being a patient with *dysautonomia*. There can never be enough talking and sharing thoughts, helping one another, learning, listening and hearing, in a support group. Taking the initiative to begin one and follow through is a major commitment, but with many rewards.

Chronic illnesses of course differ, but the social psychological effects on the patient, family, and caregivers are very similar. A chronic illness is forever. It changes lifestyles, personal relationships, goals, and vocational choices. Chronic illness is long-term and rarely curable, and so there is a baseline "constancy of illness." The sense of health and vibrancy most people expect is no more.

The need to learn "coping techniques" from others becomes imperative. Patients with chronic illness need reliable guidance—understandable, clear, compassionate, and practical. In any chronic illness there are usually at least two people to care for—the patient and the caregiver. Including the caregiver, significant other, or family members is most important. All have needs and issues.

Conquering long-term problems is best not done alone.One of the best sources of help is a support group. Successful support groups can become an invaluable entity in assisting family and friends. Participants in support groups learn quickly from one another. Professional facilitators help accomplish even more.

What is a Support Group?

A support group is a regularly scheduled, informal gathering of people whose lives are directly affected by the caregiving needs of another. Members benefit from the peer acceptance and recognition of their common concerns and are grateful for the wisdom, insight, and humor of people in the same situation.

Assuming you understand your medical diagnosis, you can put your energy into learning how to cope through support groups – listening and becoming educated by others with the illness. Support groups are also a safe place to be heard and to listen and to understand symptoms and treatments. Support groups offer understanding on how to "reinvent yourself," how to work with your healthcare team, how to communicate better with family and caregivers, and how to acquire effective strategies for daily living.

The support group may be in the best position to help patients with chronic illnesses, their thoughts and concerns regarding relationship issues, how to work with their physicians, understanding the role of the caregiver and accepting the challenge of change.

Many physicians have come to recognize the value of caregiver and care recipient support groups. Many questions regarding daily living and what to expect are answered within the group. Today, physicians, social workers, rehabilitation specialists, neuropsychologists, and others refer many patients to a recognized support group. One is the NDRF Support and Outreach Program ("Program").

Informal support groups generally are created by one or more individuals dealing with a care recipient with a common illness, or category (e.g., kids with special needs) that decide they need to reach out and to share with others, ultimately to help themselves. It doesn't take special training, but it does take effort, dedication and some ingenuity. You will also find it to be one of the most rewarding things one can do.

Support groups offer opportunities to learn from one another and to share pain and joy. A support group can be a lifesaver as well as an ally, friend, and confidant.

If you wish to learn more about becoming a support group leader or member, contact sglevy@ndrf.org.

Social Security and Disability

We thank attorney Frank W. Levin for his assistance in this chapter.

Understanding what it takes to be eligible for Social Security disability can be confusing. This chapter will try to help sort through some of the confusion. It is intended for general information and should not be taken as legal advice about your specific situation. Your right to benefits depends on all of the facts and circumstances of your particular claim. For convenience sake, all of the varied forms of autonomic dysfunction will simply be referred to as POTS.

> *This chapter gives general information and not specific legal advice.*

The Social Security Administration (SSA) administers two disability benefit programs. Each of these programs provides cash benefits and health insurance coverage. One program is called SSDI and the other is called SSI.

SSDI stands for Social Security Disability Insurance and is also referred to as RSDI (Retirement Survivors and Disability Insurance), as DIB (Disability Insurance Benefits) and as Title II.

SSI stands for Supplemental Security Income. It is also known as Title XVI. Sometimes you can be eligible for benefits under both programs. This is called a "concurrent eligibility." SSDI and SSI both have "medical" and "non-medical" (economic) eligibility requirements. In general, the medical requirements are the same. We'll get to them later.

For now we're only going to talk about some of the "non-medical" requirements.

The word "Insurance" in SSDI's name tells you that it is something like an insurance policy. In order to be eligible, you not only have to be disabled, you have to be "insured" at the time you became disabled. In order to be insured, you must have paid certain minimum amounts into Social Security during your lifetime and in the ten years before you became disabled (like the "premium" you pay to be covered by car insurance). It is important to note that you need not be insured at the time you apply for benefits, only at the time you became disabled. SSI is basically for people who have not paid enough into Social Security to be insured for SSDI benefits.

SSDI benefits depend on how much you have earned and paid into Social Security. In the year 2000, the average monthly benefit is about $750.00 with the maximum monthly benefit at about $2,000.00. Minor children or a dependent spouse may be eligible for additional benefits of up to one-half of your benefit under SSDI.

In 2000, SSI's maximum monthly benefit is $512.00. There are neither minor children nor dependent spouse benefits under SSI. (If a child is receiving SSI it is because he or she is disabled.) Some states pay an additional benefit to people who receive SSI.

Disabled people who apply for, and are awarded, SSDI benefits do not receive any payments for the first five months of their disability. But benefits can be paid retroactively for up to 12 months prior to the date on which you filed your claim if you have already been disabled for five months by then. SSI benefits cannot be paid any further back than the month after the month in which you filed your claim.

SSDI recipients are eligible for Medicare two years after the first month for which they receive a cash benefit. In SSDI, eligibility for Medicaid is dependent on financial criteria. SSI recipients are usually eligible for Medicaid.

Since SSDI is an insurance program, there is no limit on the amount of "unearned" income (such as interest, dividends, rent), you and your spouse may receive, the amount of "earned" income your spouse may receive or the amount of assets the two of you have. In contrast, since SSI is an "means-tested" program, there are limits on how much income and assets you and your spouse may have.

Under both SSDI and SSI, if you earn income at what SSA calls the "substantial gainful activity" (SGA) level, you are not eligible for benefits. SGA is currently

$700.00 per month. You are not ineligible for SSDI or SSI just because you are earning a few hundred dollars per month despite your disability. However, it is not enough that you are earning less than $700.00 per month; there must be medical evidence that you are not able to do so. In the SSI program, $65.00 per month of earnings are disregarded; after that SSI payments are reduced $1.00 for every $2.00 earned.

The length of time and the amount of paperwork your claim will require depends on how far you have to appeal it. There are potentially four levels of decisions inside SSA:
1. Initial Decision
2. Reconsideration Decision
3. Administrative Law Judge (ALJ) Decision
4. Appeals Council Decision.

In addition, there are potentially three levels of appeal in the federal courts.
1. United States District Court
2. Circuit Court of Appeals
3. United States Supreme Court

Filing a new application is not the same as appealing a decision. You might lose some benefits, or not qualify for any benefits if you file a new application instead of appealing.

You start the application process by calling SSA's no-toll number, 1-800-772-1213. Tell them that you want to file a claim for disability. Explain that you want to do this by phone rather than going to an SSA office. They will schedule a telephone conference for you. (We'll talk about the paperwork you'll need a couple of paragraphs from now.) If the operators tells you that you're ineligible because you're no longer insured, ask her what your "date last insured" (DLI) is. If you think you were already disabled by your DLI, tell her politely and firmly that you want to file a claim alleging that you were disabled before that date.

After filing an application for benefits, you will receive an initial decision. The initial decision is usually issued about 120 days after your application is received. If your claim is approved, you will get a Notice of Award. If it is denied, you will get a Notice of Disapproved Claim, which will tell you what you must do to appeal and how long you have to do it. Your first appeal is called a Request for Reconsideration.

The reconsideration decision is usually issued about 90 – 120 days after the request for reconsideration is filed. If your claim is approved, you'll get a Notice of Award, if not you'll get a Notice of Reconsideration. (About 85% of the claims are denied at the reconsideration level). Again, the notice will tell you how and when to appeal. Your next appeal is called a Request for Hearing.

There is more variation in how long it takes a case to come up for hearing than at the two previous levels. In some parts of the country, the hearing is held about 90 days after the request for hearing is filed. In other places it is 180 days or even longer. There is also a lot of variation in how long after the hearing it takes to receive a written decision – anywhere from a few weeks to several months. If the claim is approved, you will receive a Notice of Decision – Fully (or Partially) Favorable and a Decision. Approximately 60% of the claims that are appealed to the hearing level are approved, although there is a significant difference from Judge to Judge. The Decision will only indicate whether you won or not. If you won, you will later get a Notice of Award that states the amount of your monthly benefit and past-due benefits. If you lose, you will receive a Notice of Decision – Unfavorable and a Decision. The Notice will again tell you how and when to appeal. Although further appeals are possible, that's beyond the scope of this chapter.

In the application process, the first papers you will have to complete are an "Application" a "Disability Report" and medical authorizations. The Application for Disability Insurance Benefits (SSDI) and the Application for Supplemental Security Income (SSI) both give SSA biographical information, such as your name, Social Security number, and date of birth. Beyond that, the two Applications ask different kinds of questions since the "non-medical" eligibility requirements are different in the two programs.

The Disability Report is usually the most important single paper you will complete. It is your chance to tell SSA what your disabling condition is, when it became disabling, how it prevents you from working, and what activities you can and can't do with your disability. It is also your chance to tell SSA who your doctors have been. (If your insured status has expired, you may have to list doctors from years ago to establish that you were already disabled by that time.) Finally, it's your chance to tell SSA about your education and work experience, since these may determine whether there is still work you can do.

For the appeal process following a Notice of Disapproved Claim, you will have to complete a Request for Reconsideration and a Reconsideration Disability Report. If you want to appeal the reconsideration decision, you have to complete a Request for Hearing and a Claimant's Statement. Your answers on any of the forms can trigger a request for others forms, such as a Vocational Report, a Work Activity Report, and Activities of Daily Living Questionnaire or other papers SSA needs to decide your claim.

Every form you fill out must be taken very seriously.

SSA isn't just making "Small Talk" about your daily activities and your symptoms. It will use your answers to decide if you're disabled.

The actual rules SSA uses to decide whether you are disabled involve not only your physical and mental limitations, but your age, education, work experience and transferability of skills. This is because disability is a medical and <u>vocational</u> concept under the Social Security Act.

SSA uses three sets of rules to apply the medical and vocational factors to the evaluation of disability. These rules are called the "five-part sequential analysis", the "Listing" and the "Grids". The sequence of questions works like this:

1. Is the claimant currently engaged in <u>substantial gainful activity</u> (SGA)? If "yes," the claim is denied. If "No" go to Step 2.
2. Is the claimant's impairment or combination of impairments <u>severe</u> enough to significantly limit the ability to do basic work activities? If "Yes," go to Step 3. If "No," the claim is denied.
3. Does the claimant have an impairment or combination of impairments, which <u>meets</u> or <u>equals</u> the <u>Listings</u> of Impairments? If "Yes," the claim is approved. If "No," go to Step 4. (We will use the disorder known as POTS as our example).
    a.) There is no Listing for POTS. Therefore, a claimant with POTS can't "meet" a Listing.
    b.) Arguably, POTS may "equal" another Listing, for example, the syncope and near-syncope in POTS may be equivalent in duration and severity to a cardiovascular Listing for recurrent arrhythmias.
4. Does the claimant have an impairment or combination of impairments, which prevents previous relevant <u>work</u>? If "Yes," go to Step 5. If "No," the claim is denied.

5. Can the claimant, given her residual functional capacity and her age, education and past work experience perform any <u>other work</u>, which exists in substantial numbers in the national economy? If "Yes," the claim is denied. If "No," the claim is approved.

   a) In order to determine whether the claimant can do other work, SSA first decides her/his maximum exertional (strength) level.

   b) SSA then uses the "Grid" for that strength level (sedentary, light or medium).

   c) The combined effect of the claimant's strength, age, education, skill level and transferable skills determine whether she/he is presumably "disabled" or "not disabled".

   d) Finally, SSA considers the effect of non-strength limitations (fatigue, dizziness, nausea, etc.) on the ability to work.

Because there is, as yet, no listing for *POTS* or most *dysautonomias* and because much of the disability is invisible, many claimants with *POTS* will have to go all the way to an ALJ hearing. However, if you do a good job explaining your symptoms and their effect on your daily activities to your doctor, you stand an excellent chance of convincing SSA that you are disabled because you simply cannot work eight hours per day, five days per week on a sustained basis.

Children and Dysautonomia

One of the greatest fears parents face is having a child with a debilitating, life-altering, or life-threatening illness. Concern about their child's health becomes paramount.

The family with an ill child has boundaries set by the illness. It is not just the child that must learn to live and cope with the illness. The entire family must learn to adjust their lives to accommodate an ill child.

Will we need to relocate? Can we afford the medical bills? Will one of us need to quit working to be home with the child? Do we dare leave for vacation? Will the school accommodate our child's needs? These are some of the questions many young families face when a child suffers from a *dysautonomia.*

Dyautonomias are "Invisible."

Unfortunately, *dysautonomias* can be "invisible" to an outsider. This means that in addition to other challenges, there is the sense of need to "prove" the child is not just "faking it." Comments from family, friends, and sometimes even the child's doctor can be unhelpful or hurtful.

Keep in mind that if these comments upset you, they're likely to upset your child! This is when a parent needs to become the child's advocate. Take time to learn about your child's disorder. Educate yourself and your child about their condition. Make it special time! Ask your child questions. Learn your child's fears, goals, concerns, and ambitions. If your child is concerned over things that you as a parent can't help them with, it may be a good time to talk to a counselor.

We don't want our children to become fearful of every symptom that they may be experiencing, but at the same time if a new symptom arises they need to feel comfortable bringing it to your attention. Create a "Comfort Zone."

It's also important to learn about Federal and State programs that help families and individuals who suffer from disabilities.

The NDRF would like to acknowledge the National Information Center for Children and Youth with Disabilities for the following information. Each year, the National Information Center for Children and Youth with Disabilities (NICHCY) receives thousands of requests from families and professionals for information about special education and related services for children and youth with disabilities. This News Digest has been developed to answer many of the questions and concerns that families and professionals have when they contact NICHCY.

IDEA and Its Regulations

You should know the mandates and requirements of the Individuals with Disabilities Education Act Amendments of 1997 (IDEA), because it may apply to children with disabilities arising from *dysautonomia.*

This document is the federal law that supports special education and related services programming for children and youth with disabilities. Because States base their programs upon the law and its final Federal regulations, it is helpful for you to read and become familiar with the law itself. To obtain a copy of the law (called the statute) or the final Federal regulations, contact: Superintendent of Documents, U.S. Government Printing Office, Attn: New Orders, P.O.B. 371954, Pittsburgh, PA 15250-7954. Charge orders may be telephoned to: (202) 512-1800. For a copy of the statute, state that you are requesting a copy of Public Law 105-17, the Individuals with Disabilities Education Act Amendments of 1997. To obtain a copy of the final Federal regulations, request the latest copy of the IDEA's regulations: Code of Federal Regulations: Title 34; Education; Part 300-399. There will be a minimal charge for both of these documents.

This chapter discusses parts of the Individuals with Disabilities Education Act

Both of these documents are also available on the Internet at the Web site of the Office of Special Education Programs (OSEP) at the U.S. Department of Education. OSEP's Web address is: www.ed.gov/offices/OSERS/IDEA/index.html. Another useful Web site for obtaining these materials is the OSEP-funded IDEA Partnership Projects at: www.ideapractices.org/lawandregs.htm.

The major **purposes of the IDEA** are: (a) to ensure that all children with disabilities have available to them a "free appropriate public education" that emphasizes special education and related services designed to meet their unique needs and prepare them for employment and independent living; (b) to ensure that the rights of children and youth with disabilities and their parents are protected; (c) to assist States, localities, educational service agencies, and Federal agencies to provide for the education of all children with disabilities; and (d) to assess and ensure the effectiveness of efforts to educate children with disabilities.

Under the law, a **free appropriate public education** (FAPE) means special education and related services that: (a) are provided to children and youth with disabilities at public expense, under public supervision and direction, and without charge; (b) meet the standards of the State Education Agency (SEA), including the requirements of the IDEA; (c) include preschool, elementary school, or secondary school education in the State involved; and (d) are provided in keeping with an individualized education program (IEP) that meets the requirements of law.

The regulations for IDEA define a "child with a disability" as including a child (a) who has been evaluated according to IDEA's evaluation requirements; (b) who has been determined, through this evaluation, to have one or more of the disabilities listed below; and (c) who, because of the disability, needs special education and related services. The disabilities listed by IDEA are: mental retardation; a hearing impairment, including deafness; a speech or language impairment; a visual impairment, including blindness; serious emotional disturbance (hereafter referred to as emotional disturbance); an orthopedic impairment; autism; traumatic brain injury; other health impairment; a specific learning disability; deaf-blindness; or multiple disabilities.

For children ages 3 through 9, a "child with a disability" may include, at the discretion of the State and the local educational agency (LEA), and subject to certain conditions, a child who is experiencing developmental delays, as defined by the State and as measured by appropriate diagnostic instruments and procedures, in one or more of the following areas: physical development; cognitive development; communication development; social or emotional development; or adaptive development; and who needs, for that reason, special education and related services. From birth through age 2, children may be eligible for services through the Infants and Toddlers with Disabilities Program of the IDEA.

Special education is defined as instruction that is specially designed, at no cost to you as parents, to meet your child's unique needs. Specially designed instruction means adapting the content, methodology, or delivery of instruction: to address the unique needs of your child that result from his or her disability, and to ensure your child's access to the general curriculum so that he or she can meet the educational standards that applies to all children within the jurisdiction of the public agency. Special education can include instruction conducted in the classroom, in the home, in hospitals and institutions, and in other settings. It can include instruction in physical education as well. Speech-language pathology services or any other related service can be considered special education rather than a related service under State standards if the instruction is specially designed, at no cost to the parents, to meet the unique needs of a child with a disability. Travel training and vocational education also can be considered special education if these standards are met.

Special education instruction can be provided in a number of settings, such as: in the classroom, in the home, in hospitals and institutions, and in other settings. Public agencies must ensure that a continuum of alternative placements is available to meet the needs of children with disabilities. This continuum must include the placements just mentioned (instruction in regular classes, special classes, special schools, home instruction, and instruction in hospitals and institutions) and make provision for supplementary services (such as resource room or itinerant instruction) to be provided in conjunction with regular class placement.

Unless a child's IEP requires some other arrangement, the child must be educated in the school he or she would attend if he or she did not have a disability. Special education instruction must be provided to students with disabilities in what is known as the least restrictive environment, or LRE. Both the IDEA and its regulations have provisions that ensure that children with disabilities are educated with nondisabled children, to the maximum extent appropriate. The IDEA's LRE requirements apply to students in public or private institutions or other care facilities. Each State must further ensure that special classes, separate schooling, or other removal of children with disabilities from the regular educational environment occurs only if the nature or severity of the disability is such that education in regular classes with the use of supplementary aids and services cannot be achieved satisfactorily.

Related services are defined in the regulations as transportation and such developmental, corrective, and other supportive services as are required to assist a child with a disability to benefit from special education. Related services may include: speech-language pathology and audiology; psychological services; physical therapy and occupational therapy; recreation, including therapeutic recreation; early identification and assessment of disabilities in children; counseling services, including rehabilitation counseling; orientation and mobility services; and medical services for diagnostic or evaluation purposes only; school health services; social work services in schools; parent counseling and training. The list of related services identified in the IDEA's regulations is not intended to be exhaustive and could include other developmental, corrective, or support services if they are required to assist a child with a disability to benefit from special education.

You can learn more about Federal and State Disability programs by contacting the following:

NICHCY National Information Center for Children and Youth with Disabilities, P.O. Box 1492, Washington, DC 20013-1492, Phone:1-800-695-0285 or (202) 884-8200, Fax: (202) 884-8441, e-mail: nichcy@aed.org.

U.S. Department of Education OSERS/NIDRR Room 3431, FB6 Washington, DC 20202, Phone: (202) 205-5633, website: www.ed.gov, e-mail: david_keer@ed.gov.

The National Council on Disability, website: www.ncd.gov. A Guide To Disability Rights Laws is available at http://www.ncd.gov/newsroom/publications/disabilityrights.html.

It is also important to become familiar with your **State special education law.** The IDEA is a Federal law and, as such, provides minimum requirements that States must meet in order to receive Federal funds to assist in providing special education and related services. Your State law and regulations may go beyond the Federal requirements, and it is important to know their specifics. You may want to contact your State Department of Education, Office of Special Education, and ask for a parent handbook on special education.

Glossary

123I-metaiodobenzylguanidine (123I-MIBG) *A particular type of radioactive drug that is used to visualize sympathetic nerves such as in the heart.*

6-[18F]Fluorodopamine *A drug that is the catecholamine, dopamine, with a fluorine atom attached that is a radioactive isotope called a positron emitter. Positron-emitting fluorodopamine is used to visualize sympathetic nerves such as in the heart.*

-A-

Acetylcholine *A particular chemical that functions as the chemical messenger of the parasympathetic nervous system.*

ADH (Abbreviation for antidiuretic hormone).

Adrenal, adrenal gland *Glands near the tops of the kidneys that produce steroids such as cortisol and catecholamines such as adrenal.*

Adrenaline *The same as epinephrine.*

Adrenal medulla *The "marrow," or core, of the adrenal gland.*

Adrenoceptors *Specialized proteins in cell membranes of various tissues that bind to the catecholamines norepinephrine (noradrenaline) or epinephrine (adrenaline), resulting in changes in the state of activity of the cells.*

Adrenomedullary hormonal system *The part of the autonomic nervous system where epinephrine is released from the adrenal medulla.*

Aldosterone *The main sodium-retaining steroid produced in the adrenal gland.*

Alpha-1 adrenoceptors *A particular type of adrenoceptors that is prominent in blood vessel walls. Stimulation of alpha-1 adrenoceptors in blood vessel walls causes the vessels to tighten.*

Alpha-2 adrenoceptor blocker *A drug that blocks alpha-2 adrenoceptors.*

Alpha-2 adrenoceptors *A type of adrenoceptor that is present on particular cells in the brain, in blood vessel walls, in several organs, and on sympathetic nerve terminals.*

Alpha-adrenoceptors *One of the two types of receptors for norepinephrine (noradrenaline) and epinephrine (adrenaline).*

Alpha-methylDOPA (Aldomet™) *A drug that resembles levodopa and is an effective drug to treat high blood pressure.*

Amphetamines *Drugs that share a particular chemical structure that causes decreased appetite, increased attention, decreased sleep, and behavioral activation.*

Amino acid *A particular type of chemical that contains an amino chemical group and a carboxylic acid chemical group and is a "building block" of proteins.*

Anemia *A decreased amount of red blood cells. Anemic patients look pale and feel tired.*

ANS (Abbreviation for autonomic nervous system)

Antidiuretic hormone (ADH). *Same as vasopressin.*

Arterial blood sampling *Obtaining blood from a large blood vessel that moves blood away from the heart.*

Arterial pressure *The blood pressure in an artery.*

Artery *A large blood vessel that carries blood from the heart. Arteries (with the exception of the arteries to the lungs) carry oxygen-rich blood at high pressure.*

Arteriole *Like "twigs" of the arterial tree, the arterioles are tiny arteries that carry blood from the heart. The overall amount of constriction of arterioles is the main determinant of the total resistance to blood flow in the body. Constriction of arterioles therefore increases the blood pressure, just like tightening the nozzle increase the pressure in a garden hose.*

Asphyxiation *Loss of consciousness from lack of breathing, such as in suffocation.*

Aspiration *Inhalation of a foreign body into the airway.*

Auto-immune autonomic failure *A form of autonomic failure associated with an "attack" of the immune system on a part of the autonomic nervous system.*

Autonomic *Referring to the autonomic nervous system.*

Autonomic function testing *Testing of one or more functions of the autonomic nervous system.*

Autonomic Myasthenia *Nickname for a form a chronic autonomic failure associated with an antibody to the acetylcholine receptor responsible for transmission of nerve impulses in ganglia.*

Autonomic nerve supply *The amount of autonomic nerve fibers and terminals in a tissue or organ.*

Autonomic nervous system (ANS) *The body's "automatic" nervous system, responsible for many automatic, usually unconscious processes that keep the body going.*

AVP (Abbreviation for arginine vasopressin).

Axon reflex *A type of reflex where stimulation of nerves going towards the brain leads directly to a change in nerve activity towards a nearby site.*

-B-

Baroreceptor reflex *A rapid reflex where an increase in blood pressure sensed by the brain leads to relaxation of blood vessels and a decrease in heart rate.*

Baroreceptors *Stretch or distortion receptors in the walls of large blood vessels such as the carotid artery and in the heart muscle.*

Baroreflex *The same as baroreceptor reflex.*

Baroreflex Failure *An unusual disorder where the baroreceptor reflex fails, resulting in variable blood pressure and orthostatic intolerance.*

Benign Prostatic Hypertrophy (BPH) *Long-term enlargement of the prostate gland that does not result from a cancer.*

Benzodiazepine *A type of drug with a particular chemical structure that causes sedation, an anti-anxiety effect, relaxation of skeletal muscle, and decreased seizure activity.*

Beta-1 adrenoceptors *One of the three types of beta-adrenoceptors, prominent in the heart muscle.*

Beta-2 adrenoceptors *One of the three types of beta-adrenoceptors, prominent in blood vessel walls in skeletal muscle, in the heart muscle, and on sympathetic nerve terminals.*

Beta-3 adrenoceptors *One of the three types of beta-adrenoceptors, prominent in fatty tissue.*

Beta-Adrenoceptor blocker *A type of drug that blocks one more types of beta-adrenoceptors.*

Beta-Adrenoceptors *One of the two types of receptors for the norepinephrine (noradrenaline) and epinephrine (adrenaline).*

Bethanecol (Urecholine™) *A drug that stimulates some receptors for acetylcholine, mimicking some of the effects of stimulating the parasympathetic nervous system.*

Blood glucose *The concentration of the important metabolic fuel, glucose (dextrose), in the blood.*

Blood pressure *The pressure in arteries. Systolic blood pressure is the maximum pressure while the heart is beating, and diastolic blood pressure is the minimum pressure between heartbeats.*

Blood volume *The total volume of blood in the body. Most of the blood volume is in veins.*

BPH (Abbreviation for benign prostatic hypertrophy)

Brainstem *The lower part of the brain, located just above the spinal cord. The brainstem includes the hypothalamus, midbrain, pons, and, just at the top of the spinal cord, the medulla oblongata.*

-C-

Caffeic acid *A particular chemical found in coffee beans that is not caffeine.*

Caffeine *A chemical found in high concentrations in coffee beans.*

Carbidopa *A drug that inhibits the conversion of L-DOPA (levodopa) to dopamine. Because carbidopa does not enter the brain from the bloodstream,* carbidopa blocks the conversion of L-DOPA to dopamine outside the brain.

Cardiac output *The amount of blood pumped by the heart in one minute.*

Catechols *Chemicals with a structure that includes two adjacent hydroxyl groups on a benzene ring. The catecholamines norepinephrine (noradrenaline), epinephrine (adrenaline), and dopamine are catechols, as are the non-catecholamines levodopa and carbidopa in Sinemet™.*

Catecholamine *A member of an important chemical family that includes adrenaline.*

Catecholamines *Norepinephrine (noradrenaline) epinephrine (adrenaline), and dopamine.*

Cell membrane norepinephrine transporter (NET) *The transporter responsible for "recycling" of norepinephrine back into sympathetic nerves.*

Central nervous system *The brain and spinal cord.*

Central Sympathetic Hyperactivity *A condition where there is an increase in the rate of sympathetic nerve traffic in the body as a whole.*

Cerebellar *Referring to the cerebellum.*

Cerebellar atrophy *A decrease in size of the cerebellum, a part of the brain.*

Cerebellum *A part of the brain, located above and behind the brainstem, that plays important roles in coordination of movement and the sense of orientation in space.*

Cerebrospinal fluid (CSF) *The clear fluid that bathes the brain and spinal cord.*

Chiari malformation *An anatomic abnormality where part of the brainstem falls below the hole between the brain and spinal cord.*

Chronic autonomic failure *Long-term failure of the autonomic nervous system.*

Chronic fatigue syndrome *A condition where the patient has a sense of persistent fatigue for more than six months, without an identified cause.*

Chronic orthostatic intolerance *Long-term inability to tolerate standing up.*

Clearance *The volume of fluid cleared of a substance in one minute.*

Clonidine *A drug that stimulates alpha-2 adrenoceptors in the brain, in blood vessel walls, and on sympathetic nerve terminals. Clonidine decreases release of norepinephrine from sympathetic nerves and decreases blood pressure.*

Clonidine suppression test *A test based on effects of clonidine administration on blood pressure and plasma levels of chemicals such as norepinephrine (noradrenaline).*

Common faint *The same as neurocardiogenic syncope.*

Compensatory activation *A situation where failure of one effector system compensatorily activates another effector system, allowing a degree of control of a monitored variable.*

Constipation *Infrequent and difficult bowel movements.*

Coronary arteries *The arteries that deliver blood to the heart muscle.*

Coronary artery disease *A disease where the coronary arteries become narrowed or blocked by fatty deposits and thickening of the walls.*

Cranial nerves *The twelve nerves that come through holes in the skull from the brainstem and go to many organs, from the eyes to the gastrointestinal tract.*

-D-

d-Amphetamine *The dextro- mirror image form of amphetamine.*

DBH (Abbreviation for dopamine-beta-hydroxylase)

Dehydration *Abnormal lack of water in the body.*

Delayed orthostatic hypotension *A fall in blood pressure after prolonged standing.*

Denervation supersensitivity *Increased sensitivity of a process as a result of loss of delivery of a chemical messenger to its receptors that normally mediate the process.*

Dextro-amphetamine (Same as d-amphetamine)

Diabetes *A disease state with excessive volume of urination and excessive water intake. Diabetes mellitus results from lack of insulin effects in the body. Diabetes insipidus results from lack of antidiuretic hormone (vasopressin) in the body.*

Diagnosis *A decision about the cause of a specific case of disease.*

Dihydrocaffeic acid *A particular chemical that is a breakdown product of caffeic acid.*

Distress *A form of stress that is consciously experienced, where the individual senses an inability to cope, attempts to avoid or escape the situation, elicits instinctively communicated signs, and activates the adrenal gland.*

DOPA decarboxylase (DDC, LAAAD) *The enzyme responsible for conversion of L-DOPA to dopamine in the body.*

Dopamine-beta-hydroxylase (DBH) *The enzyme responsible for conversion of dopamine to norepinephrine in the body.*

Dysautonomia *A condition where a change in the function of the autonomic nervous system adversely affects health.*

-E-

Ephedrine *A particular drug that acts in the body as a sympathomimetic amine.*

Epinephrine (adrenaline) *The main hormone released from the adrenal medulla.*

EPI (Abbreviation for epinephrine)

Erectile impotence *Impotence from failure to have or sustain erection of the penis.*

Ergotamine *A particular drug that constricts blood vessels.*

Erythropoietin *A hormone that stimulates the bone marrow to produce red blood cells.*

Extravasation *Leakage of fluid from blood vessels into the surrounding tissues.*

-F-

Fainting *Relatively rapid loss of consciousness that is not caused by heart disease.*

False-positive test *A positive test result when the patient does not actually have the disease.*

Familial Dysautonomia (FD) *A rare inherited disease that features abnormalities in sensation and in functions of the autonomic nervous system.*

FBF (Abbreviation for forearm blood flow)

FD (Abbreviation for Familial Dysautonomia)

Fenfluramine *A particular drug that acts in parts of the nervous system where serotonin is the chemical messenger.*

Florinef™ (Brand name for fludrocortisone)

Fludrocortisone (Florinef™) *A type of artificial salt-retaining steroid drug.*

Fluorodopamine *A drug that is the catecholamine, dopamine, with a fluorine atom attached. The fluorine atom can be a type of radioactive isotope called a positron emitter. Positron-emitting fluorodopamine is used to visualize sympathetic nerves such as in the heart.*

Forearm blood flow (FBF) *The rate of inflow of blood into the forearm, usually expressed in terms of blood delivery per 100 cc of tissue volume per minute.*

Forearm vascular resistance (FVR) *The extent of resistance to blood flow in the forearm blood vessels.*

FVR (Abbreviation for forearm vascular resistance)

-G-

Galvanic skin response (GSR) *A physiological change in the ability of the skin to conduct electricity, due to a change in the amount of sweat.*

Ganglia *Plural of ganglion.*

Ganglion *A clump of cells where autonomic nerve impulses are relayed between the spinal cord and target organs such as the heart.*

Ganglion blocker *A type of drug that inhibits the transmission of nerve impulses in ganglia.*

Glucose *One of the body's main fuels. The same as dextrose.*

GSR (Abbreviation for galvanic skin response) *A rapid increase in electrical conduction in the skin as a result of an increase in production of sweat.*

-H-

Heart failure *A condition where the heart fails to pump an amount of blood for the tissues of the body.*

Hormone *A chemical released into the bloodstream that acts at remote sites in the body.*

HR (Abbreviation for heart rate)

Hyperadrenergic Orthostatic Intolerance *A condition where an inability to tolerate standing up is combined with signs or symptoms of excessive levels of catecholamines such as epinephrine (adrenaline).*

Hyperdynamic Circulation Syndrome *A condition where the rate and force of the heartbeat are abnormally increased.*

Hypernoradrenergic Hypertension *Long-term high blood pressure associated with increased release of norepinephrine from sympathetic nerve terminals.*

Hypertension *A condition where the blood pressure is persistently increased.*

Hypoglycemia *A condition where there is an abnormally low blood glucose level.*

Hypothermia *A condition where there is an abnormally*

low body temperature.

-I-

Impotence *Inability to have erection of the penis or ejaculation of semen.*

Inappropriate Sinus Tachycardia *Excessive fast heart rate because of excessively fast firing of the heart's pacemaker in the sinus node.*

Incontinence *Sudden involuntary urination or bowel movement.*

Inderal™ (Brand name of propranolol)

Indirectly acting sympathomimetic amine *A type of drug that produces effects similar to those of stimulating sympathetic nerves.*

Innervation *Nerve supply.*

Insulin *An important hormone released from the pancreas that helps to control the blood glucose level.*

Intravenous saline *Physiological salt-in-water solution that is given by vein.*

Iontophoresis *A way using electricity to deliver a drug to the skin surface.*

Isoproterenol (Isuprel™)

Isoproterenol Infusion Test *A test where isoproterenol is given by vein, to see if this affects the ability to tolerate tilting or to measure the body's responses to stimulation of beta-adrenoceptors.*

Isuprel™ (Brand name of isoproterenol)

-K-

Kinky hair disease *The same as Menkes disease.*

-L-

LAAAD (Abbreviation for L-aromatic-amino-acid decarboxylase)

L-aromatic-amino-acid decarboxylase (LAAAD) *The enzyme that converts levodopa to dopamine in the body.*

L-dihydroxyphenylalanine (Levodopa, L-DOPA)

L-Dihydroxyphenylserine (L-DOPS) *A particular amino acid that is converted to norepinephrine by the action of L-aromatic-amino-acid decarboxylase.*

L-DOPA (Abbreviation for L-dihydroxyphenylalanine, the same as levodopa)

L-DOPS (Abbreviation for L-dihydroxyphenylserine)

Levodopa *The same as L-DOPA and L-dihydroxyphenylalanine.*

Lumbar puncture *A procedure where a needle is inserted into the lower back, such as to sample cerebrospinal fluid.*

-M-

Ma huang *Chinese name for an herbal remedy that is ephedrine*

MAP (Abbreviation for mean arterial pressure)

Mean arterial pressure (MAP) *The average blood pressure in the arteries.*

Menkes disease *A rare inherited disease of copper metabolism that causes death in early childhood.*

Methylphenidate (Ritalin™) *A particular drug in the family of amphetamines.*

Midodrine (Proamatine™) *A particular drug that can be taken as a pill and constricts blood vessels by way of* stimulation of alpha-adrenoceptors, used commonly in the treatment of orthostatic hypotension and orthostatic intolerance.

Military antishock trousers (MAST) suit *A type of inflatable trousers that decreases pooling of blood in the legs.*

Mineralocorticoid *A type of steroid that causes the body to retain sodium.*

Monoamine *A type of biochemical that contains a component called an amine group. Serotonin and adrenaline are monoamines.*

Moxonidine *A particular drug that decreases blood pressure by decreasing sympathetic nerve traffic.*

MSA (Abbreviation for Multiple System Atrophy)

Multiple System Atrophy (MSA) *A progressive disease of the brain that includes failure of the autonomic nervous system.*

Mutation *A rare genetic change, like a "typo" in the genetic encyclopedia.*

Myocardium *Muscle tissue of the heart.*

-N-

NE (Abbreviation for norepinephrine)

Nerve terminal *The end of a nerve fiber, from which chemical messengers are released.*

NET (Abbreviation for cell membrane norepinephrine transporter)

NET Deficiency *A rare cause of orthostatic intolerance resulting from decreased activity of the cell membrane norepinephrine transporter.*

Neurally Mediated Syncope *A condition that includes sudden loss of consciousness from a change in the function of the autonomic nervous system.*

Neurasthenia (Same as neurocirculatory asthenia).

Neurocardiogenic Syncope (Same as Neurally Mediated Syncope).

Neurochemical *A chemical released from nervous tissue.*

Neurocirculatory Asthenia *A condition closely related to chronic fatigue syndrome that features exercise intolerance without identified cause, described mainly in medical literature from the former Soviet Union.*

Neuroimaging tests *Tests based on visualizing the nervous system.*

Neuropathic POTS *A form of postural tachycardia syndrome (POTS) thought to result from local or patchy loss of sympathetic nerves.*

Neuropharmacologic *A type of drug effect that acts on nervous tissue or mimics chemicals released in nervous tissue.*

Neurotransmitter *A chemical released from nerve fibers or terminals that produces effects on other cells nearby.*

Nicotine *A chemical in tobacco that stimulates a particular type of receptor for the chemical messenger acetylcholine.*

Nicotinic receptor *One of the two types of receptors for the chemical messenger acetylcholine.*

Nitroglycerine *A particular drug that relaxes walls of veins in the body.*

Non-selective beta-adrenoceptor blockers *A type of drug that blocks all types of beta-adrenoceptors.*

Norepinephrine (noradrenaline) *The main chemical messenger of the sympathetic nervous system, responsible for much of regulation of the cardiovascular system by the brain.*

Normal saline *A dilute solution of sodium chloride (table salt) that has the same concentration as in the serum.*

-O-

Orthostasis *Standing up.*

Orthostatic hypotension *A fall in blood pressure when a person stands up. This can be defined by a fall in systolic blood pressure of 20 mm Hg or more or a fall in diastolic blood pressure of 5 mm or more when the person stands up.*

Orthostatic intolerance *An inability to tolerate standing up, due to a sensation of lightheadedness or dizziness.*

Orthostatic tachycardia *An excessive increase in pulse rate when a person stands up.*

-P-

Pacemaker *A device that produces electrical impulses in the heart.*

PAF (Abbreviation for Pure Autonomic Failure)

Palpitations *A symptom where the patient notes a forceful, rapid heartbeat or a sensation of the heart "flip-flopping" in the chest.*

Panic disorder *A condition that features a rapid buildup of fear or anxiety that the patient cannot control.*

Parasympathetic nerve traffic *The rate of traffic in parasympathetic nerves.*

Parasympathetic nervous system *One of the two branches of the autonomic nervous system, responsible for many "vegetative" functions such as gastrointestinal movements after a meal.*

Parasympathetic neurocirculatory failure *Failure to regulate the heart rate appropriately, such as during normal breathing or in response to the Valsalva maneuver.*

Parkinson's disease *A nervous system disease of the brain that produces slow movements, a form of limb rigidity called "cogwheel rigidity," and a "pill-roll" tremor that decreases with intentional movement. Other features of Parkinson's disease include a mask-like facial expression, stopped posture, difficulty initiating or stopping movements, and small handwriting.*

Parkinson's disease with orthostatic hypotension *Parkinson's disease with a fall in blood pressure when the patient stands up.*

Parkinsonian *Having one or more features of Parkinson's disease.*

Parkinsonian form of MSA *A form of multiple system atrophy that includes one or more features of Parkinson's disease.*

Partial dysautonomia (Same as Neuropathic POTS)

Peristalsis *Gastrointestinal movements such as after a meal that move digested material.*

PET scanning (Abbreviation for positron emission tomographic scanning)

Phen-Fen *Two drugs, phentermine and fenfluramine, prescribed together to decrease appetite and promote weight loss.*

Phentermine *A particular drug that acts in the body as a sympathomimetic amine.*

Phenylalanine *A particular amino acid*

Phenylephrine (Brand name Neo-Synephrine™) *A particular drug that constricts blood vessels by stimulating alpha-1 adrenoceptors.*

Phenylketonuria (PKU) *A disease of children that results from lack of activity of a particular enzyme, phenylalanine hydroxylase, resulting in a toxic buildup of phenylalanine in the body.*

Phenylpropanolamine (PPE) *A particular drug that acts in the body as a sympathomimetic amine.*

Pheo (slang for pheochromocytoma)

Pheochromocytoma *An abnormal growth that produces the catecholamines norepinephrine (noradrenaline) or epinephrine (adrenaline).*

Physiological *Referring to a body function, as opposed to a body part.*

Plasma *The part of the blood that is left after anti-coagulated blood settles or is centrifuged (spun at a high rate in a tube).*

Plasma epinephrine level *The concentration of epinephrine (adrenaline) in the plasma.*

Plasma norepinephrine level *The concentration of norepinephrine (noradrenaline) in the plasma.*

Polymorphism *A genetic change that is not as rare as a mutation but not so common as to be considered normal.*

Positron emission tomographic scanning (PET scanning) *A type of nuclear medicine scan where a positron-emitting form of a drug is injected, and particular parts of the body become radioactive, with the radioactivity detected by a special type of scanner called a PET scanner.*

Positron emitter *A chemical that releases a special type of radioactivity called positrons.*

Postganglionic nerves *Nerves from the ganglia that deliver signals to nerve terminals in target tissues such as the heart.*

Post-prandial hypotension *An abnormal fall in blood pressure after eating.*

Postural Tachycardia Syndrome (POTS) *A condition where the patient has a long-term inability to tolerate standing up, along with an excessive increase in pulse rate in response to standing.*

Potassium *An important element found in all cells of the body.*

POTS (Abbreviation for Postural Tachycardia Syndrome)

Power spectral analysis of heart rate variability *A special type of test based on changes in the heart rate over time.*

PPE (Abbreviation for phenylpropanolamine)

Preganglionic nerves *Nerves of the autonomic nervous system that come from cell bodies in the spinal cord and pass through the ganglia.*

Presyncope *A feeling of near-fainting.*

Proamatine™ (Brand name of midodrine)

Procrit™ (Brand name of erythropoietin)

Progressive Supranuclear Palsy *A type of neurological syndrome with particular abnormalities of gaze.*

Propranolol (Brand name Inderal™) *A drug that is the classical non-selective beta-adrenoceptor blocker.*

Provocative test *A test designed to evoke an abnormal response of the body.*

Pseudephedrine (Sudafed™) *A particular drug that acts in the body as a sympathomimetic amine.*

Pure Autonomic Failure (PAF) *A form of long-term failure of the autonomic nervous system where there is no clear evidence for degeneration of the brain.*

-Q-

QSART (Abbreviation for Quantitative Sudomotor Axon Reflex Test)

Quantitative Sudomotor Axon Reflex Test (QSART) *A type of test of autonomic nervous system function based on the ability of drugs to evoke sweating.*

-R-

Radiofrequency ablation *Destruction of a tissue by applying radiofrequency energy, which burns the tissue.*

Receptors *Special proteins in the walls of cells that bind chemical messengers such as hormones.*

Renin System Failure

Renin-Angiotensin-Aldosterone system *A system that plays an important role in maintaining the correct amount of blood volume and sodium in the body.*

Respiratory sinus arrhythmia *The normal changes in pulse rate that occur with breathing.*

Ritalin™ (Brand name of methylphenidate) *A particular drug that resembles amphetamine.*

-S-

Salivation *Formation of spit.*

Salivary glands *Glands responsible for releasing saliva.*

Serotonin *A chemical messenger in a family called monoamines. Catecholamines such as adrenaline are also monoamines.*

Shy-Drager syndrome (multiple system atrophy with sympathetic neurocirculatory failure) *A form of nervous system disease where different pathways of the brain degenerate and the patient has a fall in blood pressure during standing, because of failure of the sympathetic nervous system.*

Sinemet™ (Brand name of levodopa, or L-DOPA)

Sinus node *The pacemaker area of the heart that normally generates the electrical impulses resulting in a coordinated heartbeat.*

Sinus node ablation *Destruction of the sinus node in the heart, usually as a treatment for excessively rapid heart rate.*

Skin sympathetic test (SST) *A type of test of the sympathetic nervous system based on the ability of various drugs or environmental manipulations to increase secretion of sweat.*

Sodium *An important chemical element found in all body fluids.*

Somatic nervous system. *The somatic nervous system is the main way the body deals with the "outside world," by way of its main target organ, skeletal muscle.*

Smooth muscle cells *The type of muscle cells in the heart and in blood vessel walls.*

SSRI (Abbreviation for selective serotonin reuptake inhibitor) *SSRIs block one of the main ways of inactivating and recycling the chemical messenger, serotonin. This increases delivery of serotonin to its receptors in the brain. SSRIs are used to treat depression, anxiety, and other psychiatric or emotional problems.*

SST (Abbreviation for skin sympathetic test)

Stereoisomer *A mirror image structure of a chemical.*

Strain gauge *A testing device that sensitively measures stretch.*

Stress *A condition where the brain senses a challenge to physical or mental stability that leads to altered activities of body systems to meet that challenge*

Striatonigral degeneration *A form of nervous system disease where the patient seems to have Parkinson's disease but does not respond well to treatment with levodopa.*

Stroke volume *The amount of blood pumped by the heart in one heartbeat.*

Sudafed™ (Brand name of pseudephedrine)

Sympathetic innervation *The supply of nerve fibers and terminals in a tissue or organ.*

Sympathetic nerve terminals *Endings of sympathetic nerves, from which the chemical messenger, norepinephrine (noradrenaline) is released.*

Sympathetic nerve traffic *Nerve impulses in sympathetic nerve fibers.*

Sympathetic nerves *Nerves of the sympathetic nervous system.*

Sympathetic nervous system *One of the two branches of the autonomic nervous system, responsible for many "automatic" functions such as constriction of blood vessels when a person stands up.*

Sympathetic neurocirculatory failure *Failure of regulation of the heart and blood vessels by the sympathetic nervous system.*

Sympathetic neuroimaging *Visualization of the sympathetic nerves in the body.*

Sympathetic vasoconstrictor tone *The status of constriction of blood vessels as a result of traffic in sympathetic nerves.*

Sympathoadrenal system (also called sympathico-adrenal system or sympathoadrenomedullary system) *A name for the sympathetic nervous system and adrenomedullary hormonal system acting as a unit.*

Sympathomimetic amine *A type of drug that acts in the body like stimulation of the sympathetic nervous system.*

Sympathotonic orthostatic intolerance *Inability to tolerate standing up that is associated with excessive activity of the sympathetic nervous system.*

Syncope *Sudden loss of consciousness due to decreased flow of blood to the brain.*

Syndrome *A set of symptoms that occur together.*

Systolic blood pressure *The peak blood pressure while the heart is pumping out blood.*

-T-

TH (Abbreviation for tyrosine hydroxylase)

Thermoregulatory sweat test (TST) *A test based on the ability of the patient to produce sweat in response to an increase in environmental temperature.*

Tilt-table testing *A test where the patient is tilted on a platform, to assess the ability of the patient to tolerate and respond appropriately to standing up.*

Tomographic scans *A type of scan where the body is visualized in slices.*

Total peripheral resistance *The total amount of resistance to blood flow.*

Tremor *Involuntary shaking.*

Trimethaphan (Arfonad™) *A particular type of drug that blocks chemical transmission in ganglia.*

Trimethaphan infusion test *A test where trimethaphan is given by vein, to assess the effects on blood pressure.*

Tyrosine hydroxylase (TH) *An important enzyme required for production of the catecholamines dopamine, norepinephrine (noradrenaline), and epinephrine (adrenaline) in the body.*

-U-

Uptake-1 *Uptake of norepinephrine and related chemicals by way of the cell membrane norepinephrine transporter, such as uptake into sympathetic nerves.*

-V-

Vagal parasympathetic outflow *Traffic in the vagus nerve, a main nerve of the parasympathetic nervous system.*

Valsalva maneuver *A type of maneuver where the person blows against a resistance or strains as if trying to have a bowel movement, resulting in an increase in pressure in the chest and a decrease in the ejection of blood by the heart.*

Vascular resistance *Resistance to blood flow.*

Vasoconstriction *Tightening of blood vessel walls.*

Vasodepressor syncope (Same as Neurocardiogenic
Syncope and Neurally Mediated Syncope).

Vasopressin (the same as antidiuretic hormone) *A
hormone released from the pituitary gland at the
base of the brain that stimulates retention of water
by the kidneys and increases blood pressure by
constricting blood vessels.*

Ventricles *The main pumping chambers of the heart. The
right ventricle contains blood pumped by the heart
to the lungs. The left ventricle contains blood
pumped by the heart to the rest of the body. The left
ventricular myocardium is the main pumping muscle
of the heart.*

Venous return *Return of blood to the heart by the veins.*

Vesicular monoamine transporter (VMAT) *A particular
type of protein in the walls of storage vesicles that
transports chemicals such as norepinephrine into
the vesicles.*

VMAT (Abbreviation for the vesicular monoamine
transporter)

-Y-

Yohimbe bark *A naturally occurring form of yohimbine
that is available as an over-the-counter herbal
remedy.*

Yohimbine *A drug that blocks alpha-2 adrenoceptors in
the brain, in blood vessel walls, and on sympathetic
nerve terminals.*

Yohimbine challenge test *A test where yohimbine is
administered and the effects are measured on blood
pressure and plasma levels of chemicals such as
norepinephrine (noradrenaline).*